NURSING RESEARCH

AN INTRODUCTION

NURSING RESEARCH

AN INTRODUCTION

Mildred O. Hogstel, R.N., C., Ph.D.

Professor of Nursing
Harris College of Nursing
Texas Christian University

Nancy C. Sayner, R.N., D.N.Sc.

Associate Dean and Associate Professor of Nursing
Harris College of Nursing
Texas Christian University

McGRAW-HILL BOOK COMPANY

New York   St. Louis   San Francisco   Auckland   Bogotá
Hamburg   Johannesburg   London   Madrid   Mexico   Montreal   New Delhi
Panama   Paris   São Paulo   Singapore   Sydney   Tokyo   Toronto

NURSING RESEARCH
An Introduction

1 2 3 4 5 6 7 8 9 0 DOCDOC 8 9 8 7 6

ISBN 0-07-029375-9

This book was set in Times Roman by Kachina Typesetting Inc.
The editor was Sally J. Barhydt;
the cover was designed by Laura Stover;
the production supervisor was Phil Galea.
Project supervision was done by Cobb/Dunlop Publisher Services Incorporated.
R. R. Donnelley & Sons Company was printer and binder.

Library of Congress Cataloging in Publication Data

Hogstel, Mildred O.
  Nursing research.

  Includes bibliographies and index.
  1. Nursing—Research. I. Sayner, Nancy C. (Nancy
Carol) II. Title. [DNLM; 1. Nursing. 2. Research.
WY 20.5 H716n]
RT81.5.H65 1986   610.73'072   85-13244
ISBN 0-07-029375-9

To our parents . . . and

To nursing students and
practicing professional nurses
who seek new answers
to old questions and
who propose new questions
which need answers.

CONTENTS

PREFACE

Research is becoming increasingly important in the continuing growth and development of nurses and nursing. Although there has been a core of nurse researchers who have been working diligently to increase the theoretical base for nursing for some time, the majority of nurses have not been prepared in their educational programs to appreciate, evaluate, and utilize research findings.

One of the purposes of this book, therefore, is to reach those nurses who have had little or no experience with the research process. At this point in the history of nursing, research is emerging at all levels in nursing practice settings. Nurses are beginning to be more interested in learning about research. Nursing research committees are expanding in all clinical agencies. Nurses are attending workshops on research in greater numbers.

The primary purpose of this book is to introduce the nurse to the research process in the clearest way possible. The most basic elements of the research process are included. The two major goals of the book are to help the nurse: (1) understand how to read, evaluate, and apply research findings in the clinical setting and (2) learn how to identify clinical problems and devise a simple research plan to study those problems.

This book is intended for baccalaureate degree nursing students at all levels, whether the research content is integrated throughout the curriculum or taught in a specific research course. The book is also intended for the practicing nurse who may or may not have had research content and experience in the basic nursing program. In any case, the book is written for the nurse who has had little or no background or experience in research.

Section I introduces the reader to the basic elements of research. A brief history of the development of research in nursing also is included. The major components of the research process are included in Section II for the reader who wishes to initiate a research study. These include a discussion of the research purpose, problem, and question, the literature review, methodological approaches, and the collection and analysis of data. Section III emphasizes the application of research findings in the clinical area by helping the nurse learn how to read and evaluate research reports. Guidelines are also given that will help the beginning researcher learn how to write a research proposal and research report. The final Section IV gives suggestions on how to initiate research in the clinical setting.

The authors hope that the readers of this book will begin to discover, as we have, that research is not only vigorous, stimulating, and thought-provoking, but that it can also be fun and very rewarding personally. Seeing nurses at various levels experience the excitement of developing and expanding their own ideas through the research process is very satisfying. It is hoped that more and more nurses will have these same experiences.

ACKNOWLEDGEMENTS

Appreciation is expressed to Hugh Macdonald, Wendy Gottlieb, and Sandy Echt of the Mary Couts Burnett Library, Texas Christian University, for their suggestions and review of Chapter 4.

We are grateful to the Literary Executor of the late Sir Ronald A. Fisher, F.R.S., to Dr. Frank Yates, F.R.S., and to Longman Group Ltd., London, for permission to reprint Table III. from their book *Statistical Tables for Biological, Agricultural and Medical Research* (6th Edition, 1974) in Chapter 7.

Appreciation is expressed to Dr. Majorie Caballero, Assistant Professor of Marketing, Hankamer School of Business, Baylor University, Waco, Texas, for her review of Chapter 7.

We also want to thank our typists, Susan Moore, Donna Taylor, Joyce A. Valentine, and Carolyn Wood for their patience, flexibility, and expertise. A thank you is also extended to Andrew Haskett and Rob Devoe for their assistance in the development of some of the tables and figures.

Finally, we want to express appreciation to many of our former students, who have shown us how well beginning researchers are able to understand and implement research studies based on their own ideas and identified problems.

Mildred O. Hogstel

Nancy C. Sayner

NURSING RESEARCH

AN INTRODUCTION

THE BASIC ELEMENTS
OF RESEARCH

CHAPTER 1

THE BASIC FACTORS SURROUNDING RESEARCH

Research is frequently thought of by many individuals as a lofty, complex, and impractical endeavor which has little or no bearing on the everyday activities of the average person. Research is also considered by some individuals to be an activity confined entirely to the laboratory setting under a highly controlled environment. These impressions of research reflect misunderstandings and incorrect information about the value and purpose of research as well as the potential research offers. The purpose of this chapter is to describe the basic factors surrounding research in relation to the what, why, how, when, and where of research and to provide an overview of the following chapters.

The standard of living we enjoy and the quality of life that we experience are a direct result of the advances gained through research. Most of what is considered the essentials of daily living have resulted from individual or group efforts in research. Whether these essentials are household appliances, modes of communication, means of transportation, food preparation, or the health status one experiences, each one has been derived from the efforts of research.

Research has improved the health status of all. Advances in medical science and technology, pharmacology, and preventive health care measures have provided a level of health care and longevity that was not considered possible only a few decades ago. Organ transplants and test tube babies are areas of recent medical research. Research in nursing has included the value of preoperative teaching, client decision-making, maternal and child attachment, the role of the nurse practitioner, and the means of promoting client compliance with prescribed medical regimens. The benefits of research to society are immeasurable.

THE WHAT OF RESEARCH

Research has been defined in a number of different ways. Formally, research is defined as a scientific search or inquiry involving an investigation or experimentation aimed at the discovery and interpretation of facts, or the practical application of new or revised theories.[1] Although this definition is comprehensive, a more functional definition indicates that research is a systematic way of thinking involving a sequential number of steps which reflect the highest level of scientific inquiry. To conduct research, therefore, a system of thinking is required which involves a number of steps in sequence. Based on this more functional definition, research becomes more realistic as it relates to many of our ongoing activities of daily living that require a systematic and organized manner of thinking.

To accomplish a certain number of tasks each day, planning is required. Usually those individuals who accomplish these tasks assess them according to priority and within a time frame. For example, to attend classes, prepare a written assignment, review content for a midsemester examination, and engage in study time, as well as attend to personal considerations and allow time for recreational activities, a systematic and organized plan is required. Preparing for a day's assignment in the clinical area when caring for a number of patients also dictates a systematic way of thinking which involves a plan of priority setting and a time frame. Performing a sterile dressing change for a patient requires the same thought process in planning both from an organizational stance and a time frame. Thus, those activities experienced in everyday life frequently require a plan of systematic thinking involving a sequence of steps and share some of the similar and basic characteristics of research. Research is conducted in all disciplines in a similar way. Whether research is conducted in psychology, chemistry, or nursing, the purpose and the process involved do not significantly differ.

The terms *nursing research* and *research in nursing* need to be made clear. The former refers to research that has as its subject the care process and the problems that are encountered in the practice of nursing such as hygiene maintenance, rest, sleep, nutrition, relief from discomfort, counseling, health education, and rehabilitation. *Research in nursing* refers to research on the profession of nursing, and includes studies on practitioners and the characteristics of their practices, utilization costs, administration, career patterns, and the educational levels of nurses and nursing students.[2,3,4]

THE PROCESS OF RESEARCH

Research begins with an interest in a particular area of nursing. A survey of the literature that relates directly to that area of interest is conducted. A problem statement is then identified and subsequently a research question is conceived. Following the conceptualization of the research question, a number of sequential steps are developed that reflect the process of research. The final step of the research process culminates with the research findings and the possible identification of further areas for research. Although the number of steps in the research process vary, the sequence of steps is of utmost importance, and it is always followed when the research is being developed or proposed. Whether the research process is developed according to eight steps or sixteen steps, two major phases of the process may be identified. These two phases, although interrelated to some extent, are the *conceptualization,* or *thinking phase* and the *factual,* or *doing phase.*[5] Frequently the steps are combined, reordered, or repeated, resulting in a variation in the number of steps. The research process may, therefore, be developed according to many different formats. Two examples of different formats which include both the *conceptualization phase* and the *factual phase* are depicted in Table 1–1.

The examples in Table 1–1 represent two different formats or outlines of the sequential steps inherent in the research process.[6] The two phases reflect those activities concerned with the *thinking* processes of research and those activities related to the *doing* activities of research. In both Examples I and II, the conceptualization, or thinking phase represents activities that must be cognitively developed, explored, and analyzed. The second phase of Examples I and II represents the factual, or doing phase of the research process in which implementation of a number of activities is required. The second phase of the research process, therefore, includes those activities that can be correlated with actualizing or implementing steps that reflect movement and direction. Although the factual, or doing phase incorporates the steps associated with doing activities, this phase does not negate critical thinking.

THE WHY OF RESEARCH

The significance of research to nursing cannot be overemphasized and is directly related to the image of nursing as a profession. Professions are recognized by society as

TABLE 1–1
STEPS OF THE RESEARCH PROCESS

Example I	Example II
Conceptualization Processes (Thinking Phase)	
Formulating and delimiting the problem	Problem identification (development and hypothesis)
Reviewing the literature	
Developing a conceptual-theoretical framework	Literature review
Formulating the hypothesis	Conceptual framework development
	Definition of terms
Factual Processes (Doing Phase)	
Selecting a research design	Methodological approach (design)
Specifying the population	Data collection plan
Operationalizing and measuring the research variables	Sample selection
	Data analysis
Conducting a pilot study and making revisions	Identification of further areas for research
Selecting the sample	
Collecting the data	
Organizing the data for analysis	
Analyzing the data	
Interpreting the results	
Communicating the findings	

Example I taken from Polit, Denise F. and Hungler, Bernadette P., *Nursing Research: Principles and Methods*, 2d ed., Lippincott, Philadelphia, 1983. Used with permission.

possessing a unique set of skills and knowledge, incorporating a defined body of knowledge relevant to specified activities, and being regulated by a code of conduct and ethics endorsed by its membership.[7] Professions, in addition, are often characterized as being endorsed by the community and possessing a commitment to defined goals and objectives.

A major way nursing can develop a defined body of knowledge and, subsequently, improve its professional image is through research. *Research provides the scientific foundation for professional nursing practice.* For decades nurses were satisfied to solve problems or answer questions that arose in practice by intuition, supposition, or trial and error methods. In addition to these means of solving problems or answering questions in clinical practice, nurses practiced according to what they had learned from their educational preparation and their experiences as well as what was viewed appropriate by persons in positions of authority. Although these means of answering questions, solving problems, and implementing nursing practice were satisfactory at one time, they are no longer acceptable. Today the provision of quality care to educated and sophisticated consumers requires that the activities of professional nursing practice be validated through scientific inquiry.[8]

THE HOW OF RESEARCH

The how of research refers to the methods or methodological approaches used to conduct research. Research is conducted through several different methodological approaches. The most appropriate methodological approach is dependent upon the way in which the problem statement or research question is conceptualized. Thus, the conceptualized problem statement or research question is of utmost importance, as it dictates the appropriate methodology.

Research questions are developed through the processes of thought. They may be characterized by either a *deductive* way of thinking or an *inductive* way of thinking. *Deductive* thinking involves taking statements known to be true and deducing other statements.[9] Deductive thinking involves the identification of general and known statements about a certain phenomenon and subsequently deriving other statements from them. Thus, the statement "if A = B and B = C, then A = C" denotes deductive thinking. An example of deductive thinking in nursing is as follows:

Anxious patients experience nausea and vomiting preoperatively.
Cardiovascular patients are anxious.
Therefore, cardiovascular patients will experience nausea and vomiting preoperatively.

Inductive thinking is different in that it involves a synthesis of ideas and thoughts in which factors that pertain to a specific phenomenon or situation are identified and related to other situations.[10] Inductive thinking, thus, refers to the combining of various factors found in one particular situation that are, subsequently, generalized or applied to another situation. An example of inductive thinking in nursing is as follows:

Patients/clients undergoing microvascular neurosurgical bypass for the prevention of stroke experience five phases in their process of decision making: threat, trust, holding, contemplation, and compliance. Patients undergoing similar surgical procedures involving prevention will also experience these five phases in their process of decision making.

Major Categories of Research

Based on the thought processes of deductive and inductive thinking and their relation to research, three major categories of research may be identified: experimental, quasi-experimental, and field research studies, *or* nonexperimental research. Each of these major categories may be identified on a continuum of deductive to inductive thinking. The continuum of deductive thinking to inductive thinking and the three major categories of research as well as their respective characteristics are shown in Figure 1–1.

Types of Research

Types of research which include descriptive, exploratory, explanatory, historical, and survey derive from one of the three major categories of research. The type of research that is derived results from the way in which the research question is posed and where the research question falls on the continuum in relation to the characteristics of each major category of research. Thus, if the research question is stated deductively, yet the implementation of the research requires a real world setting, the type of research that results involves characteristics reflective of both ends of the continuum and will fall somewhere between the experimental and the field research study or the nonexperimental end of the continuum. For example, consider the following research question:

> Does the administration of ice chips every four hours to the semicomatose brain-injured patient in the Surgical Intensive Care Unit increase the heart rate as reflected on the electrocardiogram monitor?

Several characteristics of the question can be identified: (1) the research question is deductive in nature as it suggests that through observations associated with an un-

FIGURE 1–1
The research continuum.

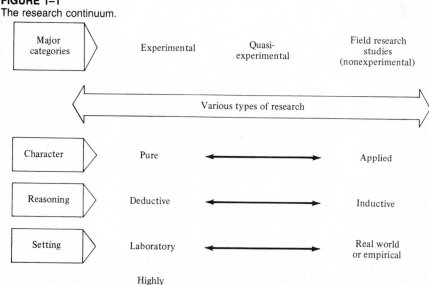

derstanding of physiology a relationship is anticipated between the administration of ice chips and the heart rate, which are considered variables, (2) the research question requires the use of a real world setting in contrast to a highly controlled setting similar to a laboratory, and (3) the research question suggests that the findings have application.

Based on the above characteristics, the research question would fall on the continuum somewhere between the research categories of experimental and field research studies, or nonexperimental research, in the area of quasi-experimental research. The type of research would basically be descriptive (see Chapter 5).

THE WHEN OF RESEARCH

When is research in nursing indicated? Research is indicated when solutions to problems are needed, when questions arise in nursing practice, or when direction in the practice of nursing is indicated. Because research involves the highest degree of scientific rigor, is time consuming, and inappropriate for solving problems encountered in one's everyday activities, the problems identified for research must be carefully assessed. Researchable problems that suggest direction in nursing practice or contribute to the existing body of nursing knowledge are particularly significant. Examples of researchable problems in nursing include the following:

1 What are the differences in the infection rate of three types of meatal or Foley catheter regimens?

2 Do the stress levels of nursing staff on the acute care units differ from the stress levels of nursing staff on the general units as measured by a selected scale?

3 Does the introduction of a structured preoperative teaching plan decrease the hospitalization stay of patients undergoing coronary artery bypass surgery?

4 Is the incidence of phlebitis higher in those patients in Intensive Care Units who receive intravenous care every 48 hours than those patients who receive intravenous care every 24 hours?

5 What are the perceptions of a panel selection process for hospital staff positions as viewed by the panel members and the respective candidates?

As noted above, each researchable problem is stated as a question. Researchable problems may also be stated in a declarative form in their initial development; however, once the researchable problem has been finalized the question format is more appropriate, as it has the virtue of posing the problem in a more direct way.[11] For purposes of this text and in lieu of the preferences of different authors, researchable problems will be used interchangeably with research questions.

THE WHERE OF RESEARCH

The solution to problems or answers to questions are not confined to any particular area of nursing. Research is needed in all areas of nursing to provide direction for nursing practice. Whether nursing involves direct patient care in the inpatient setting, the follow-up activities associated with postnatal home care, or the provision of an educational experience to adult learners, questions can frequently be found or problems encountered. Research in nursing, therefore, is an appropriate endeavor anywhere.

PROBLEM-SOLVING AND RESEARCH

In contrast to problems that may be studied by research efforts in the clinical setting, problems and questions often arise that are appropriate for solution on a problem-solving basis. Problem-solving, like research, involves a systematic way of thinking and a sequence of steps. In problem-solving, the problem is identified, the alternatives to the problem solution are considered, an identified alternative is selected and implemented, and the results are evaluated.[12] Problem-solving, in addition to possessing characteristics similar to research, has similar characteristics to the nursing process and the decision-making process, as each of these processes involves the identification of a problem and is followed by a sequence of steps. Problem-solving is also considered a scientific way of thinking, but in contrast to research, the thinking that is required in problem-solving is used to solve problems that occur in our everyday activities. Problem-solving is generally a short-term process and research involves a longer period of time. Problem-solving usually consists of four major steps, in contrast to research, which requires many more steps, as previously discussed. Scientific rigor is also considerably less in problem-solving. The aim in problem-solving is to find solutions to problems; the aim of research is not only to find solutions to problems but also to determine answers to questions, which may or may not require a specific solution but adds to or complements existing knowledge. See Table 1–2.

Examples of problems that are amenable to problem-solving include the following:

1 What is the most economical assignment system for staffing the general medical-surgical units?

TABLE 1–2
CHARACTERISTICS OF PROBLEM-SOLVING, RESEARCH, AND THEORY

Problem-Solving	Research	Theory
Identification of a problem	Identification of a problem, exploration of a question	Global exploration
Sequential steps	Sequential steps	No specific problem or question
Amenable to everyday solution	Highest level of scientific inquiry	
Scientific approach	Rigorous	Deductive and inductive
Short-term	Long-term	Some parts may be subject to research
	Deductive or inductive	Relationship of concepts
		Seeks to describe, explain, predict, or prescribe

2 What interdisciplinary services are indicated in preparation for Mrs. Smith's discharge to her home?

3 What in-service education program can be developed to increase the staff's awareness of current nursing measures for the prevention of skin breakdown?

4 What are the major nursing interventions for the care of the newborn?

THEORY AND RESEARCH

The formulation of research questions derived from either deductive or inductive thinking is directly related to the development of theory. Theory is the creative invention of a number of concepts in a relationship that seeks to describe, explain, predict, or prescribe.[13] Concepts are ideas that represent some particular phenomenon and include terms such as pain, loss, health, stress, and professionalism. Although theory is initially developed through the process of inductive thinking, deductive thinking is involved as relationships between and among the concepts are subsequently constructed to form propositions. A proposition is a statement of a relationship between two or more concepts.

Theory guides the practice of nursing by the formulation of a minimum set of generalizations that allow an explanation of the relationships among the concepts. Because theory assumes a goal orientation, it provides a tool that makes practice more efficient and effective. Although theory development in nursing has been limited in scope to date, several nursing theories are currently providing a guide to nursing practice. The following theory by King is presented as an example of a nursing theory that guides nursing practice.

> Man [*sic*] functions in *social systems* through *interpersonal relationships* in terms of *perception* which influences his *life* and *health*.[14]

The example of King's theory indicates that specific concepts have been identified and arranged in such a manner that the relationship of the concepts results in a definitive proposition.

A major purpose of theory is to guide research. Through the identification of concepts and the formulation of propositions theories provide the boundaries within which questions can be asked. Because of its global nature, theory is not subject in its entirety to research; however, parts of theory are amenable to research. Research can be implemented to validate and modify parts of theory, which in turn guides the practice of nursing.[15] Theory can be a stimulus to research endeavors, serving as a springboard to scientific advances in nursing.

SUMMARY

The five factors surrounding research can be described by answering the questions what, why, how, when, and where. Research is defined as a systematic way of thinking involving a sequential number of steps that reflect the highest level of scientific inquiry. The research process consists of two major phases that include the *conceptualization,* or *thinking phase* and the *factual,* or *doing phase.* The major purpose of conducting research in nursing is to provide quality care that is based on scientific inquiry.

The research question determines the appropriate methodology used to conduct research. Three major categories of research are experimental, quasi-experimental, and field research studies, or nonexperimental research, which can be placed on a *research continuum*. Based on the characteristics of each of the three major categories of research, various *types* of research are derived. Appropriate times to conduct research are when questions require answers, problems need solutions, or direction in nursing practice is indicated. Consistent with the appropriate times that are indicated to conduct research, all areas of nursing are potential research settings. Examples of research questions were presented to illustrate the variety of research questions that could be conceptualized.

Research, theory, and problem-solving are each distinct entities, but they share some similarities and differences. Problem-solving is short-term, and is used for the solution of everyday problems. Research, the highest level of scientific inquiry, is time-consuming, long-term, and involves more steps than problem-solving. Theory guides nursing practice and is global in nature. Theory as a whole is not subject to research, but parts of theory may be amenable to scientific inquiry through research. The distinguishing feature of problem-solving, research, and theory is the purpose for which each is intended.

QUESTIONS FOR STUDY AND DISCUSSION

1 Describe the relationship of research to one's everyday activities.
2 Explain the difference between nursing research and research in nursing.
3 Discuss the what, why, how, when, and where of research.
4 Compare and contrast problem-solving, research, and theory.
5 Differentiate between deductive thinking and inductive thinking.
6 Formulate one researchable question that reflects deductive thinking and one researchable question that indicates inductive thinking.
7 Describe the major categories of the research continuum.
8 Explain the variations in the number of steps involved in research.
9 Discuss the significance of research to the profession of nursing.
10 Develop in writing one question amenable to solution by problem-solving and one question that indicates a research approach.

REFERENCES

1 *Webster's Ninth New Collegiate Dictionary*, Merriam-Webster, Inc., Springfield, Massachusetts, 1983, p. 1208.
2 Jean R. Folta, "Conference on the Nature of Science and Nursing: Perspectives of an Applied Scientist," *Nursing Research*, vol. 17, no. 6, 1968, pp. 502–505.
3 Lucille L. Notter, "The Nature of Science and Nursing" (editorial), *Nursing Research*, vol. 17, no. 6, 1968, p. 483.
4 Susan R. Gortner, "Research for a Practice Profession," *Nursing Research*, vol. 24, no. 3, 1975, pp. 193–197.
5 Shirley S. Chater, and Marlene Kramer, *Cooperative Education in Nursing*, COGEN Tapes, 1972.
6 Denise Polit, and Bernadette Hungler, *Nursing Research: Principles and Methods*, 2d ed., Lippincott, Philadelphia, 1983, p. 55.

7 Janice R. Ellis, and Celia L. Hartley, *Nursing in Today's World: Challenges, Issues, and Trends*, 2d ed., Lippincott, Philadelphia, 1984, pp. 1–23.

8 Patricia A. Dempsey, and Arthur D. Dempsey, *The Research Process in Nursing*, Van Nostrand, New York, 1981, p. 7.

9 Fred N. Kerlinger, *Foundations of Behavioral Research*, 2d ed., Holt, Rinehart, and Winston, New York, 1973, pp. 12–13.

10 Eleanor W. Treece, and James W. Treece, Jr., *Elements of Research in Nursing*, 3d ed., Mosby, St. Louis, 1982, p. 68.

11 Kerlinger, op. cit., p. 18.

12 Treece and Treece, op. cit., pp. 53–54.

13 Ada Jacox, "Theory Construction in Nursing: An Overview," *Nursing Research*, vol. 23, no. 1, 1974, pp. 4–12.

14 Imogene King, "A Conceptual Frame for Nursing," *Nursing Research*, vol. 17, no. 1, 1968, pp. 27–30.

15 Afaf I. Meleis, *Theoretical Nursing: Development and Progress*, Lippincott, Philadelphia, 1985, p. 30.

BIBLIOGRAPHY

Andrioli, Kathleen G., and Carol E. Thompson, "The Nature of Science in Nursing," *Image: The Journal of Nursing Scholarship*, vol. 9, no. 2, 1977, pp. 32–37.

Brink, Pamela J., and Marilynn J. Wood, *Basic Steps in Planning Nursing Research from Question to Proposal*, 2d ed., Wadsworth Health Sciences Division, Belmont, California, 1983.

Chinn, Peggy L., and Maeona K. Jacobs, *Theory and Nursing: A Systematic Approach*, Mosby, St. Louis, 1983.

Dempsey, Patricia A., and Arthur D. Dempsey, *The Research Process in Nursing*, van Nostrand, New York, 1981.

Dickoff, James, and Patrica James, "A Theory of Theories: A Position Paper," *Nursing Research*, vol. 17, no. 3, 1968, pp. 197–203.

Diers, Donna, *Research in Nursing Practice*, Lippincott, Philadelphia, 1979.

Jacox, Ada, "Theory Construction in Nursing," *Nursing Research*, vol. 23, no. 1, 1974, pp. 4–12.

Krampitz, Sydney D., and Natalie Pavlovich: *Readings for Nursing Research*, Mosby, St. Louis, 1981.

Newman, Margaret A., "Nursing's Theoretical Evolution," *Nursing Outlook*, vol. 20, no. 7, 1972, pp. 449–453.

Polit, Denise F., and Bernadette P. Hungler, *Nursing Research: Principles and Methods*, 2d. ed., Lippincott, Philadelphia, 1983.

Shelley, Sonya I., *Research Methods in Nursing and Health*, Little, Brown, Boston, 1984.

Sweeney, Mary A., and Peter Olivieri, *An Introduction to Nursing Research*, Lippincott, Philadelphia, 1981.

Treece, Eleanor W., and James W. Treece, *Elements of Research in Nursing*, 3d ed., Mosby, St. Louis, 1982.

Verhonick, Phyllis J., and Catherine C. Seamon, *Research Methods for Undergraduate Students in Nursing*, Appleton-Century-Crofts, New York, 1978.

Walker, Lorraine O., "Toward a Clearer Understanding of the Concept of Nursing Theory," *Nursing Research*, vol. 20, no. 5, 1971, pp. 428–434.

CHAPTER 2

DEVELOPMENT OF RESEARCH IN NURSING

Scientific investigation is relatively new in nursing. When considering that organized nursing is less than one hundred years old, however, perhaps it is not unusual that research in the field is rather recent. In the early part of this century, nursing was concerned with initiating licensure, organizing and reviewing educational programs, and improving working conditions for nurses. Although there were some nurses doing research before 1950[1,2], the primary development of research in nursing has been since that date, with the most rapid development and expansion occurring in the 1970s and 1980s.

FACTORS AFFECTING THE DEVELOPMENT OF NURSING RESEARCH

Some of the basic factors that have affected the development of research in nursing over the past one hundred years are:

- Educational preparation for nursing
- Nursing primarily as a woman's career
- Effects of wars
- Effect of research in clinical settings

Educational Preparation for Nursing

Florence Nightingale not only started the first school of nursing in 1860 and has been considered the first dietitian, but she could also be called the first nurse researcher and a pioneer in statistics.[3] Kviz and Knafl[4] stated that "her work is characterized by the careful collection, analysis, and interpretation of the empirical evidence that she reported in her efforts to initiate social change" and that "she was a pioneer in the development and application of statistical methods to the study of social problems." This description of Nightingale is far different from the image that many people have of her.

Nightingale made numerous observations and detailed written notes about the hospital environment, patients, equipment, and supplies. Not only was she able to organize all of her observations in a systematic manner, but she also arrived at logical conclusions based on her observations. Results of her observations were utilized to influence leaders in her society who could assist in providing more humane and effective care for the sick and lonely. Nightingale was very persistent over a period of many years in planning, organizing, and recommending improved care for patients.

Schools of nursing began to develop in the United States in the 1870s.[5] The location of these schools in large hospitals connected with medical schools where students were taught by physicians influenced the type of organization, management, and control under which they functioned. Instead of using many of Nightingale's ideas as a model, these schools quickly fell under the control and supervision of the hospital boards of directors, managers, and physicians. As hospitals expanded, the emphasis in nursing was on providing more service to the hospital and preparing more nurses. According to McManus, "The need to increase the body of nursing knowledge was not completely lost sight of, yet it was pushed into the background."[6] Thus, some of the ideas and functions Florence Nightingale envisioned for nursing were lost. The traditionalism, ritualism, and hierarchy (administrators at the top and nursing students at the bottom) in hospitals affected the "training" of nurses for years. Nurses were expected to do what had been done in the past and to do what they were told without questioning those in authority or attempting to make changes.

Such an environment was not one in which an inquiring and questioning mind was encouraged. Even as late as the 1950s and 1960s, nursing students often were not encouraged to have open, inquisitive, questioning minds. Part of this was probably because the management and control of the nursing school was in a hospital setting. The traditional purpose of the hospital was (and is) to give patient care. Questioning the care given by others (physicians, nurse supervisors, and nurse instructors, for example) was just not done. Students were taught what their instructors had been taught, and they did what they were told to do. An editorial in *Nursing Outlook* in 1965 stated, "So much of what we have taught and practiced in nursing, and still do, has been based on tradition and empiricism. The development of action research should lessen our dependence on both."[7]

When nursing education began to move from a hospital-controlled environment to a university setting, there were many changes. The primary purposes of the university are to disseminate knowledge and to discover new knowledge. New knowledge is generated through the process of research. If nursing was to seek and obtain a position as an academic discipline in a university setting, research had to become one of the tools of the profession. However, there were few, if any, nurses prepared to do or teach research in the 1940s and 1950s, so as graduate programs (first master's and then doctoral programs) in nursing developed, faculty in academic disciplines other than nursing (such as psychology, education, sociology, and biology) taught research courses to nurses.

When nurse faculty members began to become prepared in research and had experience doing research, they soon taught the research and research-related courses themselves. Thus, as nurses have become prepared to perform *and* teach research, research content has gradually been added to the baccalaureate-degree nursing program, emphasized in the master's program in nursing, and become a major part of doctoral programs in nursing. The lack of doctorally prepared nurses before the 1970s, however, was another major factor that hindered the development of research in nursing. In the early 1960s there were only about 300 nurses with doctoral degrees in the United States.[8] Most of them were employed in administrative positions in nursing education or practice and were not conducting postdoctoral nursing research.

If nursing and nursing education had followed the ideas, philosophy, and organization of Florence Nightingale's school of nursing more closely than the apprentice-type programs that developed in the United States, the development of nursing and research in nursing would probably be 100 years ahead of what it is today.

Nursing Primarily as a Woman's Career

Closely related to the educational influence on research is the fact that nursing has been primarily a woman's career. Few women in the 1900 to 1940 period were encouraged to seek a university education, and there were few nursing programs in universities. Even if women had sought a baccalaureate-degree program in nursing during that time period, there would not have been any emphasis on research in their educational programs. There were few women, and especially nurses, seeking doctoral degrees (where research is a major focus) until the 1970s and 1980s. Girls were taught to be less assertive and were more willing than boys to do what they were told; therefore, they were more likely to grow up less inquisitive of the world about them.

With recent emphasis on women's liberation, more women are seeking higher education. Higher degrees in nursing include an emphasis on research. Women are learning to become more assertive through workshops on assertiveness as well as in their educational programs. Women are more likely now to stand up, speak out, and thus question past and present practices in their own lives and in nursing. An open, inquiring, and questioning mind is essential to the development of research interest and skills. Students now are encouraged to believe in their own ideas, to *question* theories, the ideas of others, and procedures as well as to *ask questions* about such content. Examples of the differences between *questioning* and *asking questions* are found in Table 2–1.

Thinking one's own thoughts and believing in those thoughts and ideas enough to dare to share them and try them out with others is important in developing an inquiring and inquisitive mind. An inquiring mind is a prerequisite to thinking through nursing problems and doing research.

Effect of Wars

Despite the drastic effects of war on human beings and the environment, wars have always produced some positive effects because of the necessity to make changes. Medicine and nursing have developed and grown because of situations that occurred as a result of war. Beginning with the Crimean War, when Florence Nightingale changed and organized the way injured soldiers were cared for despite the protests of army surgeons,

TABLE 2–1
QUESTIONING AND ASKING QUESTIONS

Content	Questioning Why or Why not?	Asking Questions What? How? When? Who?
The ratio method will be used to calculate fractional doses of days	Why? (I know an easier way)	How?
A nursing student should not witness a living will	Why not? (I am of legal age)	When?
Family members should not remain in the patient's room during certain nursing procedures	Why not? (Maybe they can help)	When?

to nurses who served near the front lines during World War I, to the changes that occurred in nursing education, ambulation, and rehabilitation as a result of World War II, nursing began to change as medicine changed. Thus, as medical treatment began to change and nurses began to practice their profession in a wider variety of settings, nurses began to make changes in their profession and their education to meet the needs and demands of society.

Effect of Research in Clinical Settings

Even though early nurse researchers were eager to try out their ideas to improve nursing care with their new knowledge and skills, other nurses often did not want to accept or assist them. Part of this reluctance was owing to their lack of knowledge about and/or experience in research. Nurses in practice settings were concerned about their patients' welfare, fearing that experimenting with nursing care would be harmful to them. Others, not prepared in a university setting where research was introduced, and/or not naturally inquisitive about problems encountered in their nursing care, believed that nursing research was not important when compared with the "hands-on" nursing practice with which they were more comfortable. Many nurses are not interested in pursuing research themselves. However, Notter,[9] an early nurse researcher, stressed that, "Every nurse has a role in nursing research, either as a principal investigator, as a participant in inquiry, or as a user of research findings in her [sic] practice."

NURSING RESEARCH EVOLVES

Figure 2–1 shows how research has evolved as the profession developed from the 1800s and on into the 1990s. After nurses first began to organize and license themselves, they began to be interested in improving educational programs in nursing. Although not considered research studies as defined today, but detailed reports of nursing education as practiced and proposed at that time were: (1) *A Curriculum Guide for Schools of Nursing,* prepared by the Education Committee of the National League of Nursing Education, first published in 1917,[10] and (2) the Goldmark Study of a select number of nursing schools across the United States at the time.[11]

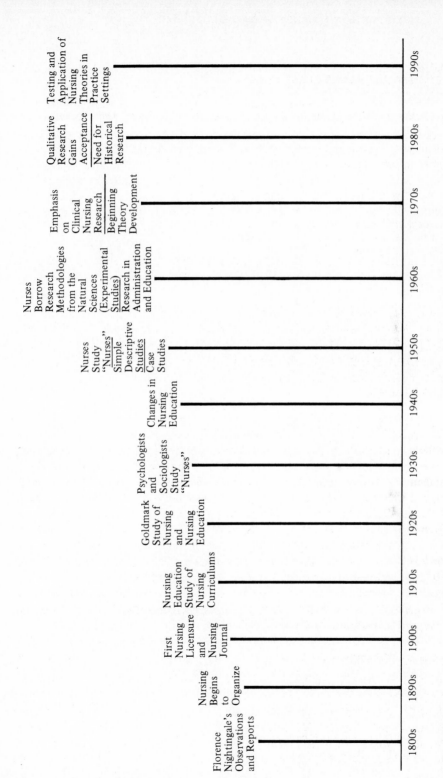

FIGURE 2–1
The historical evolvement of nursing research.

17

As research in the behavioral and social sciences (especially psychology and sociology) expanded, some of these researchers studied the role of *nurses* (not *nursing*) and the hospital environment.[12,13]

When university-based nursing programs began to expand in the 1940s, some nurses with baccalaureate degrees obtained master's degrees in related fields and then established master's programs in nursing. At this point *nurses* began to start doing research in the *field of nursing*. Nurses in the 1950s started to study *themselves*. They studied the education, status, working conditions, and personality characteristics of nurses. In 1956, Henderson[14] noted that in most occupations more research was done on practice than on the practitioner. She identified a major concern when she said, "Why is it then, that in our field, studies on the nurse outnumber studies on the practice of nursing more than ten to one?"

Nurses also started to do some simple descriptive studies related to procedures, time and motion studies,[15] and uniforms (whether uniforms or regular dress should be worn in specific areas, such as psychiatric nursing). They eventually started to study *nursing* in the analysis of patient case studies (patient case studies having been taught in most nursing schools). There was some funding for nursing research provided by the American Nurses' Association in the 1950s,[16] and the American Nurses' Foundation, Inc. was created in 1955.[17] There was a Nursing Research Conference held at the Walter Reed Army Institute of Research in Washington, D.C., in early 1959 in an attempt to increase the knowledge of research by army nurses.[18]

The first nursing research conference sponsored by the American Nurses' Association was held in April, 1965. There were 55 nurse researchers present. The studies presented and critiqued related to nursing education, nursing students, and hospital personnel.[19] In the 1963 "Report of the Surgeon Generals' Consultant Group on Nursing," many of the recommendations related to the need to expand and fund studies in nursing.[20,21]

In an attempt to apply research methodologies learned in other academic disciplines, where they often received their doctoral degrees, some nurses began to do experimental studies in clinical settings in the 1960s.[22] One of the early problems studied was the postoperative effect of preoperative teaching on the surgical patient.[23]

In the Summer 1965 issue of *Nursing Research,* however, of the eight research articles published, only one could be identified as a clinical study. The other eight articles dealt with nurses, nursing education, or nursing students.

The 1970s brought an increased emphasis on clinical research (research related to direct patient care as opposed to research on *nurses,* nursing *education,* or nursing *management*) and research that began to form a basis for various nursing theories.

The 1980s produced more acceptance of diversity in research design and methodology as nursing has grown as a profession. Nurses prepared at the doctoral level have received their research preparation in a wide variety of educational programs where there were differing emphases. Some nurse researchers believe strongly in a deductive approach involving complex quantitative methodology and sophisticated statistical analysis. Others have been prepared to utilize an inductive approach involving qualitative methodology. These approaches will be discussed in detail in Chapter 5. While there was a period of time when nurse researchers with these differing backgrounds were not particularly accepting of different research approaches, the need for research in nursing is so great that most realistic nurse researchers now believe that all valid research approaches and methodologies should be accepted and encouraged in order for the profession to grow and develop.

There has been a limited amount of historical research in nursing, and this approach is receiving increasing emphasis in the 1980s. With the rapid expansion in the number of nursing journals, for example, nurses are less likely to be aware of all of the past and present studies on a particular topic. The availability of library computer searches, discussed in Chapter 4, should facilitate additional historical research. It would be very helpful if more nurses would seek, study, and analyze what has previously been studied and written about on a particular topic. Such studies would save time and expense, particularly for nursing students who have limited time to complete a required research project.

THE NEED FOR RESEARCH IN NURSING

The major purposes of research in nursing may be grouped into several major categories:

- Professionalism
- Development and testing of nursing theories
- Application in nursing practice and improvement of patient care

Professionalism

One of the traditional criteria of a profession is that it will expand its theoretical basis through the use of the scientific method of investigation.[24,25] If a profession is to grow, develop, expand, and improve, there must be change. Change should be made based on a reasonable rationale if it is to be effective and useful. In earlier years, there was a continuing debate about whether or not nursing was a profession. That is, the question was asked if nursing met the same criteria for professionalism as medicine and law, for example. That debate has, at last, been put to rest as higher education has become the basic preparation for professional nursing practice, continuing education becomes required for license renewal, and individual nurses and nursing become more independent and autonomous. The increasing quantity and quality of research have helped to demonstrate that nursing is a profession.

Development and Testing of Nursing Theories

There were several early nurse leaders who developed their own concepts, definitions, and/or philosophies of nursing (for example, Nightingale, Henderson, Kreuter, and Peplau).[26] Even though their ideas had some of the characteristics of nursing theories, they were not labeled as such. When more and more nurses completed doctoral study in the 1960s, however, and doctoral programs in nursing expanded in the 1970s, one of the purposes of this advanced study in nursing was to discover and develop, through nursing research, a more specific and scientific theoretical base for nursing.

Several nurse leaders have developed rather complete and complex nursing theories, and they are now in the process of being tested in the practice setting through systematic study.[27] The 1980s and 1990s will be a fascinating and interesting period of nursing as these theories are tested and new theories emerge as a result of research.

Application in Nursing Practice and Improvement of Patient Care

The ultimate goal of research is to improve the profession of nursing—nursing practice, nursing management, and nursing education—as these nursing theories and others yet to be conceived continue to be developed, tested, and refined. Not too far in the future all well-prepared nurses will be basing their nursing practice on one or more specific nursing theories that have been tested scientifically through research.

While the development and testing of these theories will be performed by nurse scholars with doctoral and postdoctoral educational preparation, nursing students and practicing nurses have a responsibility to themselves and to their profession to be aware of the development of these theories in nursing practice by reading the nursing literature and trying out and/or testing some of the components of these theories in their clinical practice.

CURRENT AND FUTURE TRENDS

Despite the slow beginning and the many factors that have hindered the development of research in nursing, the quantity and quality of research has been increasing tremendously in recent years. At a recent annual meeting of the American Public Health Association, for example, the Gerontological Section scheduled one session on gerontological nursing research for the first time. The meeting room was unexpectedly overflowing, and the presentations by doctorally prepared nurse researchers were excellent and stimulating. Although nurses have presented research findings in various nursing research seminars and workshops for years, the presentation of research findings by nurses to multidisciplinary health care groups helps to reflect how far nursing research has developed in the last few years.

Research content is now included in most baccalaureate-degree nursing programs, either as a separate course or integrated into several other courses. One of the National League for Nursing (NLN) criteria for the evaluation and accreditation of baccalaureate-degree programs states that, "The research process and its contribution to nursing is included in the curriculum."[28] In one survey of NLN-accredited baccalaureate-degree programs, Spruck[29] found that of 263 baccalaureate-degree nursing programs surveyed, 164 (62%) of them required a separate research course. She concluded that research content is required in most baccalaureate-degree nursing programs and that most schools require that students conduct a research project of some type. In a similar study, Thomas and Price[30] found that 198 of 205 baccalaureate-degree nursing programs reported that research content was included in their curriculums.

Parker and Labadie[31] have suggested that research content should be integrated into the baccalaureate-degree program *before* the senior year and that students should be encouraged to become part of ongoing research projects being conducted by faculty in the institution. They also noted that "Research and study programs at the undergraduate level abound in other disciplines." The implication is that if psychology and sociology students begin to read and study about research at the freshman and sophomore levels, why cannot research be introduced in early nursing courses?

Although it is generally agreed that research content should be at the baccalaureate level in nursing, the question seems to be what breadth and depth should be expected. Levin[32] has suggested that if expectations are too great, students may not enjoy research courses or see the value of learning about research, and thus not incorporate the concepts of research into their nursing practice. The emphasis on integration of research into all courses, including the application of research findings in clinical courses, should help students to see research as a part of the nursing process.

In the future, therefore, it is expected that baccalaureate-degree nursing graduates not only will have an appreciation for research, but also that they will have experience in utilizing and applying research findings in the clinical settings. Baccalaureate-degree graduates who seek graduate degrees will also have a good foundation for research, so that they will continue to develop and expand their research knowledge and skills at the master's and doctoral levels if desired. Often students who begin the study of a nursing problem on the baccalaureate level will continue to pursue the same problem in greater depth and breadth at the master's and/or doctoral levels. Some nurse researchers have devoted most of their time and energies over a period of many years to a specific nursing problem or question. These kinds of pursuits will eventually help to build a strong theoretical base for nursing practice.

The Future

What will be the primary focus of nursing research for the rest of this century? Probably the continued testing of evolving nursing theories. Perhaps more nurses will see the value of historical research. New designs or methodologies unique to nursing may develop. There will be an increasing amount of research in practice, education, and administration. Cluster research by small groups of nurses will increase. Increased baccalaureate and master's student involvement in faculty research projects will occur. There will be more interest in research and more research by nurses employed in practice settings. Whatever the particular emphasis, there will be an increase in research in all settings as nurses continue to seek new solutions to old problems and new concerns as they emerge.

SUMMARY

Research has been slow to evolve in nursing because of several factors. One of the reasons was the early type of educational preparation for nursing in a hospital setting where traditionalism, authority, and direct patient care were more important than the search for new knowledge that would produce change. Because nursing has traditionally been a woman's career, few women in the early 1900s sought and/or completed a university education where research is a major goal. Also, women, and especially nurses, were often expected to do as they were told, with little encouragement to question policies, procedures, and authoritative figures in their nursing educational program and nursing practice.

Wars have had a positive effect on nursing research because they have forced change. While the role of women was still subservient to authoritarian leaders, the lack of adequate nursing personnel brought about some unexpected, but positive, changes in medicine and health care in general, which opened the door to change and improvement in nursing care. Some nurses themselves have discouraged the research of other nurses either because of their lack of knowledge and/or information about research or because of their fear that research would somehow harm their patients.

Some of the first studies in nursing were in the field of nursing education. Then social scientists began to study nurses as they became interested in describing relationships and behaviors in the hospital environment. Early nurse researchers followed the trend and also studied nurses or nursing education. Eventually, as nurses began to gain expertise in various clinical specialties, they started to study nursing *practice* and clinical research was emphasized above all other. More recently, a wide range of nursing research has been developing that includes practice, education, and management.

Nursing research will continue to expand and develop into the 1980s and 1990s. Not only will the quantity and quality of research by nurse scholars increase, but even more importantly, more and more nurses will be able to evaluate and utilize research findings and thus improve their nursing practice and patient care.

QUESTIONS FOR STUDY AND DISCUSSION

1 Why is Florence Nightingale called the first nurse researcher?

2 What are *three* factors that have hindered the development of research in nursing?

3 How has the development of nursing education affected the development of nursing research?

4 What was the focus or content of the first research studies in nursing?

5 What is the relationship between research and professionalism?

6 What is the ultimate purpose of research in nursing?

7 What is the relationship between nursing research and nursing theory?

8 What type of research content and experiences should be included in the baccalaureate-degree nursing curriculum?

9 What types of research are being emphasized in the 1980s?

10 What are some future trends in nursing research?

REFERENCES

1 R. Louise McManus, "Nursing Research—Its Evolution," *American Journal of Nursing,* vol. 61, no. 4, 1961, p. 79.

2 Lucille E. Notter, "The Case for Nursing Research," *Nursing Outlook,* vol. 23, no. 12, 1975, p. 760.

3 McManus, op. cit., p. 77.

4 Frederick J. Kviz, and Kathleen Austin Knafl, *Statistics for Nurses,* Little, Brown, Boston, 1980, p. 1.

5 Josephine A. Dolan, *Nursing in Society,* Philadelphia, Saunders, 1973, p. 194.

6 McManus, op. cit., p. 77.

7 Editorial, *Nursing Outlook,* vol. 13, no. 5, 1965, p. 33.

8 *Toward Quality in Nursing, Needs and Goals,* Report of the Surgeon General's Consultant Group on Nursing, U.S. Department of Health, Education, and Welfare, Public Health Service, 1963, p. 52.

9 Notter, op. cit., p. 760.

10 *A Curriculum Guide for Schools of Nursing,* Education Committee of the National League of Nursing Education, New York, 1917.

11 *Nursing and Nursing Education in the United States,* Macmillan, New York, 1923.

12 Jack V. Buerkle, "An Exploration of Attitudes Functioning Within the Operating Room Situation," *Nursing Research,* vol. 4, no. 3, 1956, pp. 125–127.

13 *Toward Quality in Nursing, Needs and Goals,* op. cit., p. 51.

14 Virginia Henderson, "Research in Nursing Practice–When?" (editorial), *Nursing Research,* vol. 4, no. 3, 1956, p. 99.

15 Notter, op. cit., p. 760.

16 *Toward Quality in Nursing, Needs and Goals,* op. cit., p. 51.

17 R. Louise McManus, "Today and Tomorrow in Nursing Research," *American Journal of Nursing,* vol. 61, no. 5, 1961, p. 68.

18 *Report of Nursing Research Conference,* Walter Reed Army Institute of Research, Walter Reed Army Medical Center, Washington, D.C., 1959.

19 "The First American Nurses' Association Nursing Research Conference" (editorial), *Nursing Research,* vol. 14, no. 2, 1965, p. 99.

20 *Toward Quality in Nursing, Needs and Goals,* 1963, pp. 52–53.

21 Lulu Wolf Hassenplug, and Rozella M. Schlotfeldt, "Report of the Surgeon General's Consultant Group on Nursing," *Nursing Research,* vol. 12, no. 2, 1963, pp. 68–71.

22 Thelma N. Thornton, and Robert C. Leonard, "Experimental Comparison of Effectiveness and Efficiency of Three Nursing Approaches," *Nursing Research,* vol. 13, no. 2, 1964, pp. 122–125.

23 Rhetaugh G. Dumas, and Robert C. Leonard, "The Effect of Nursing on the Incidence of Postoperative Vomiting," *Nursing Research,* vol. 12, no. 1, 1963, pp. 12–15.

24 Genevieve Knight Bixler, and Roy White Bixler, "The Professional Status of Nursing," *American Journal of Nursing,* vol. 45, no. 9, 1945, pp. 730–735.

25 Abraham Flexner, "Is Social Work a Profession?" Proceeding of the National Conference of Charities and Corrections, 315 Plymouth Court, Chicago, National Conference of Charities and Corrections, 1915, pp. 576–590.

26 Karen Creason Sorensen, and Joan Luckmann, *Basic Nursing,* Saunders, Philadelphia, 1979, pp. 51–52.

27 Peggy L. Chinn, and Maeona K. Jacobs, *Theory and Nursing,* Mosby, St. Louis, 1983, pp. 180–198.

28 *Criteria for the Approval of Baccalaureate and Higher Degree Programs,* 5th ed., National League for Nursing, Council on Baccalaureate and Higher Degree Programs, September, 1983.

29 Marie Spruck, "Teaching Research at the Undergraduate Level," *Nursing Research,* vol. 29, no. 4, 1980, pp. 258–259.

30 Barbara Thomas, and Marjorie M. Price, "Research Preparation in Baccalaureate Nursing Education," *Nursing Research,* vol. 29, no. 4, 1980, p. 260.

31 Meredith L. Parker, and Georgie Conaly Labadie, "Demystifying Research Mystique," *Nursing and Health Care,* vol. 4, no. 7, 1983, pp. 383–384.

32 Rona F. Levin, "Research for the Undergraduate: Too Much, Too Soon," *Nursing Outlook,* vol. 31, no. 5, 1983, pp. 258–259.

BIBLIOGRAPHY

Bunge, Helen L., "The First Decade of Nursing Research," *Nursing Research,* vol. 11, no. 3. 1962, pp. 132–137.

Notter, Lucille, *Essentials of Nursing Research,* Springer, New York, 1983.

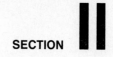

THE RESEARCH PROCESS

CHAPTER 3

THE RESEARCH PROBLEM, PURPOSE, HYPOTHESIS, AND CONCEPTUAL FRAMEWORK

Identification of the problem and formulation of the research question are the most significant and vital steps in the process of conducting research. The research question is the key to every research effort, as it provides the necessary direction for the remaining steps of the process. Research questions that are poorly conceived lack the essential ingredients that contribute to sound and well-developed research studies. Most of the major weaknesses of research studies can be directly related to problem identification or research question formulation. The purpose of this chapter is to provide the essential knowledge base to research question formulation in order that its significance in the research process can be understood and appreciated for the vital role it plays in developing and conducting research. The purpose of research, which is frequently included in the research process, the research hypothesis, and the conceptual framework are also discussed.

SIGNIFICANCE OF THE RESEARCH QUESTION

The vital role the research question plays in the research process cannot be over-emphasized. Just as problem-solving requires an accurate identification of the problem in order that alternatives may be selected and solutions identified, research questions must be formulated in exacting and precise ways to produce appropriate findings. Until it is known what is being asked, one is at a loss as to what direction is indicated, and the thinking and doing phases as discussed in Chapter 1 become meaningless. The well-developed and formulated research question, in the way it is stated, will indicate to the researcher the kind of reasoning the research question is suggesting, the type of research being contemplated, the focus of the literature review, the methodological approach, including a number of factors related to the research design, and some inclination of the anticipated answer(s) or findings. Thus, the research question provides the essential direction for the remaining steps of the research process.[1]

PROBLEM IDENTIFICATION

Problem identification is a preliminary step in formulating a researchable question. Although some researchers are able to forego the necessary thinking process of problem identification and can initially formulate the research question, most novice researchers begin the process with the identification of a problem. Only after continued refinement of the problem for research can the problem be transposed to a well-formulated research question. Problems that are potential researchable questions are found in all areas of nursing. These areas may be nursing education settings or nursing practice settings. Wherever nursing has a role potential researchable problems can be found.

For most beginning researchers, the identification of a problem that may be researchable presents a challenge. Where are these potential researchable questions and how are they formulated? What is the specific process that is involved in formulating a good researchable problem or the research question? Deciding where to start becomes a frustrating experience for those whose experience in research has been limited. However, before one can complete any project of any kind a point to begin is required.

DISCOVERY AREAS OF RESEARCHABLE PROBLEMS

To identify potential researchable problems requires that the individual be cognizant of three areas that are unique to the researcher: (1) thoughts, (2) observations, and (3) experiences. In each area of one's thoughts, experiences, or observations lie ideas for research that are potential sources of researchable problems.[2,3] Being aware and highly conscious of these areas in everyday activities facilitates the thinking process toward developing researchable questions.

Thoughts, Observations, Experiences

Thoughts about everyday experiences as a nursing student or a graduate of nursing can produce a number of problems that have the potential of meeting the criteria of a well-formulated research question. Whether those thoughts are conveyed through communication or are manifested as unexpressed ideas, few people can deny that this phenomenon occurs in their everyday lives. Experiences are also a ready source of potential researchable problems. A heightened awareness of these experiences is fertile ground for the identification of researchable questions. Observations are additionally another source for potential researchable questions. Through the senses, particularly the visual and auditory senses, problems amenable to research can be conceived. The following examples represent thoughts, observations, and experiences that can cultivate potential researchable problems.

Thought: "I wonder why admission days for our preoperative patients are always so complicated and confusing?"

Observations: "Mrs. Jones, age 84, sleeps better at night when I spend a few minutes talking with her and leave the bathroom light on."

Experiences: Dr. Cares' patients always seem to be discharged from their surgery earlier than Dr. Smith's patients.

Cues to Thoughts, Observations, Experiences

Thoughts, observations, and experiences of one's everyday activities may be manifested in several ways. These ways may be considered cues to identifying researchable problems and can be depicted according to symbolic representation (shown in Figure 3–1).

Gripes.   All too frequently complaints are expressed by others or ourselves. An expression of dissatisfaction or a gripe frequently represents an excellent place from which researchable problems can be identified. Awareness of the dissatisfaction and the understanding that these gripes, complaints, or dissatisfactions can materialize into constructive action through research may be a beginning step in identifying researchable problems.

Wish.   Often in the activities of everyday living the word *wish* comes into the conscious thought. An expression of a wish is another way or cue in which our thoughts,

FIGURE 3–1
Cues to research problem formulation.

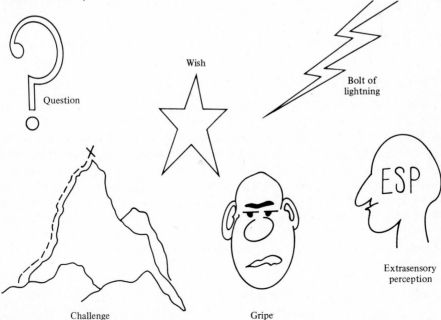

observations, and experiences may be manifested. Being cognizant of the key word *wish* often represents an area by which researchable problems can evolve.

Lightning.   Sometimes, within the arena of wondering thoughts, a flash of insight occurs in which a response is brought into our conscious experience and the words *of course* are noted. Flashes of insight also represent an area where initial thinking can be instrumental in identifying researchable problems.

Question.   Questions or thoughts reflective of a questioning nature may also play a significant role in identifying researchable problems. Often an awareness of a thought, such as "I wonder why," or "How come," begins the initial thinking process required for developing researchable problems.

Challenge.   A fifth cue that frequently derives from thoughts, observations, and experiences, and may provide the basis from which researchable problems evolve, is an inner desire or feeling expressed as a challenge. "I know I can prove this" or "I am sure there is a better way" represent thoughts or expressions of thoughts that may reflect the beginnings of identifying researchable problems. Challenges usually represent feelings and, if developed in a constructive manner, are particularly solid areas from which researchable problems can be generated.

Extrasensory Perception.   The phenomenon of extrasensory perception is, in addition, another fertile area from which researchable problems can be identified. Extrasensory perception represents a creative sense that, at times, manifests itself through cognitive insights in relation to not only researchable problem identification but also problem solution. An awareness of this cue is significant; however, few novices in research are fortunate enough to have been blessed with this attribute.

The above discussion of six cues to how thoughts, observations, and experiences may be manifested and subsequently processed to researchable problem identification indicates that even the beginning researcher has a place from which to start. One must be continually aware of these six cues, however. That *awareness* must be cultivated and consciously practiced. It basically requires a sensitizing of oneself to the way the cues are manifested. Awareness of our thoughts, our expressions, and those of whom we interact with provides the basis from which the generation of researchable problems become feasible. And because for the most part, the cues represent the individual's own thoughts, observations, and experiences, each identified researchable problem will represent the individual's own uniqueness. Thus, few identified researchable problems are exactly alike. To summarize these six significant cues to researchable problem identification the following examples are provided:

Cues	*Possible Thoughts/Expressions*
1. Gripes	"I'm sick of the way in which we must function on this unit."
2. Wish	"I wish we could determine a usable plan of care."

3. Lightning   "Of course, I should have known."
4. Question   "I wonder why this procedure is always so uncomfortable for this patient."
5. Challenge   "I know there is a better way of facilitating the patient's learning."
6. ESP   "The quality of the care these patients are receiving can be improved upon by an interdisciplinary approach."

ADDITIONAL AREAS FOR THE DEVELOPMENT OF RESEARCHABLE PROBLEMS

Other areas in which thoughts, observations, and experiences are manifested through cues and which represent ideal sites from which researchable problem identification may evolve are readings and various theories presently used in nursing.[4]

Reading

If reading is done for the purpose of enriching our knowledge base and if it is done with comprehension, it offers another source from which researchable problems may be conceived. Frequently, readings that are done prior to patient assignments generate questions in applying what has been read to the clinical experience. The accompanying experiences based upon this reading often provide the basis of questions that may assist in the development of a researchable question. Additional reading in a particular area of interest frequently provides the groundwork for developing researchable questions. Review of the literature offers additional substantive knowledge in a particular area of interest and will enhance a narrowing, or focusing, of questions consistent with the generation of researchable questions. How the review of the literature assists in problem identification is discussed in more depth in Chapter 4.

Theory

Although the profession of nursing may be considered in its infant stage as a result of the limited amount of knowledge it has generated that is specifically related to nursing, the continued development of nursing theories as well as those currently in existence offer fertile grounds for research. Parts or portions of several nursing theories are amenable to testing through research. Research efforts directed toward verifying various components of theory provide the scientific basis for that theory and substantiates the significance of the theory for professional nursing. Thus, theories provide another source from which researchable problems may be generated.

ASSESSMENT OF THE RESEARCH PROBLEM/QUESTION

Once the research problem has been formulated and refined there are several criteria by which the research problem may be assessed for its quality. The research problem, however, must first be translated into a research question. Thus, all researchable problems, once formulated, are transposed into a question format. Examples of this transformation from problem to question are illustrated in Table 3–1.

TABLE 3–1

1. Research statement/problem:
   Administration of ice chips to semiunconscious brain-injured patients in the Intensive Care Unit increases the heart rate.
   Research question*
   Does the administration of ice chips to semiunconscious brain-injured patients in the Intensive Care Unit increase the heart rate as measured by the electrocardiogram monitors?

2. Research statement/problem
   Preoperative teaching decreases the patient's anxiety level postoperatively.
   Research question*
   Does preoperative teaching of these patients undergoing coronary bypass surgery decrease the anxiety level postoperatively, as indicated by the frequency of pain medication that is requested?

3. Research statement/problem
   Meals-on-Wheels increases the wellness level of clients/patients in the home.
   Research question*
   Does the community's project of Meals-on-Wheels decrease the number and frequency of hospitalizations of homebound clients/patients?

*Note how much more concise and focused the research question becomes in the transition from research statement/problem to the research question.

To assess the researchable problem or question for its appropriateness as a well-stated research problem or question, several inquiries of that formulated research question need to be discussed. These inquiries that need to be addressed are the criteria by which well-formulated research questions are assessed.[5,6] They include the criteria of: (1) clarity, (2) significance to nursing, (3) testing feasibility, (4) measurability, and (5) relationship of variables.

Clarity

A well-formulated and well-stated researchable problem/question must be clear, concise, comprehensive, and not open to misinterpretation.[7] Thus, the researchable problem/question is stated in a manner consistent with good English composition. It communicates to the reader a question or inquiry that is clearly posed, concisely asked, easily identifiable and is able to be meaningfully understood by the reader. A well-stated researchable problem/question provides not only the researcher but others an exactness and specificity that prevents any misinterpretation. It is broad enough to include all the parameters that relate to the question, yet it is sufficiently focused and narrow to avoid ambiguity. Since both novice and experienced researchers frequently spend weeks or months developing the research problem/question and subsequently become very involved in the question, wisdom dictates the use of others to assess the research problem/question according to these five criteria.

Significance to Nursing

A second criterion for assessing well-formulated research problems/questions is to assess the question in relation to its significance to nursing. If the research problem/

question is deemed insignificant to the profession of nursing by the researcher or others, it probably is questionable if the time and energy required to be invested in conducting the research is worthwhile. If the research question can be viewed as making a *difference* to professional nursing, it probably would be a worthwhile research endeavor.

Testing Feasibility

The feasibility of testing is the third criterion by which researchable problems/questions require assessment. Is the research question amenable to testing? This criterion is directly related to methodology. The question basically asks whether or not the research can be implemented. Factors such as time, involvement, financial requirements, sample availability, and ethical considerations all need to be assessed in relation to feasibility of testing. If doubts are apparent in any of these considerations, the feasibility of testing is questionable.

Measurability

The fourth criterion for assessing researchable problems/questions is measurement.[8] Are the variables in the research question measurable? Is there some method available that would be appropriate to measure the variables? If the variables cannot be measured, then quantification or statistical significance to analyze the results or findings is impossible. Although this criterion is as important as all the other assessment criteria, the researcher may realize, simply by the way the research question is being posed, that the measurement of the variables is not appropriate to the methodological approach indicated. This fact is to be acknowledged in conducting exploratory field research studies in which the research question seeks answers from a qualitative base rather than a quantitative one. Thus, research questions that are characterized as being inductively developed and seek qualitative data may not be amenable to measurement in the usual sense of quantification (refer to Chapter 5).

Relationship of Variables

The last criterion by which researchable questions are assessed is the relationship of variables.[9] Does the research question suggest that a relationship among two or more of the variables exist? This criterion, as well as the criterion of measurability, discussed above, is of particular significance for those research questions that indicate quantification or an area developed from the deductive mode of thinking. Inductive studies do not, as their main objective, suggest a relationship of the variables.

BARRIERS TO RESEARCHABLE QUESTIONS

After the research question has been assessed as to its clarity, significance, testability, measurability, and relationship of variables, it requires an additional analysis in relation to appropriateness. The appropriateness of the research question refers to the areas of: (1) yes-no, (2) should-could, and (3) opinions.

Yes-No

Sometimes researchable problems, once transposed to the research question, and assessed according to the above criteria, can be answered simply by a yes or no. If an answer of yes or no is apparent, the research question is probably unsound and not amenable to scientific inquiry or research. Examples of yes-no research questions are as follows:

1 Does health care increase an individual's longevity?

2 Does the Headstart program for preschool-age children increase the child's readiness to learn?

The above examples of research questions suggest, based upon current knowledge, that an answer of yes would be indicated. The questions, therefore, would be a barrier, or inhibitor, or a stop to a well-developed and well-conceived research question.

Should-Could

Another barrier to a well-developed and well-conceived researchable question is the formulation of the question that indicates a should or could answer. Research questions that imply a should or a could reflect individual values and suggest subjectivity, and consequently, they lack the objectivity required of a scientific endeavor. Researchable problems and questions suggesting an individual's value system present a second barrier to well-developed research questions. An example of a should or could research question might be, "Should nursing students be required to take a course in interpersonal relationships?"

Opinion

Research questions that suggest an opinion are also considered barriers to well-developed and well-conceived researchable questions. Although opinion questions indicate a value to some extent, they frequently indicate a particular individual's position. Thus, personal beliefs are another barrier to well-developed research questions. A question such as, "Do terminally ill patients who have an option of euthanasia verbalize the dying process to a greater extent than those patients who do not have this option?" suggests a personal belief or value and lacks the scientific objectivity that is required.

A well-developed researchable question that can be answered by a yes or no, reflects a should or could stance, or indicates an opinion are definitive barriers or stops to sound researchable questions.

THE RESEARCH PURPOSE

The purpose of the research addresses the rationale of *why* the research is being proposed.[10] The problem or research question, in contrast, addresses the *what* of the research.[11] Placement of the research purpose in the research proposal or the written plan of the proposed research varies with authors.[12,13] The purpose may be included in the introduction to the research proposed or a statement that follows the research question. In either case, the purpose is a necessary step in the conceptualization, or thinking, phase discussed in Chapter 1, and it needs to be included in the sequential steps of the research process. The authors believe that the appropriate placement of the purpose in the research process lies within the introduction as a brief statement to the proposed research that reflects an explanatory characteristic consistent with the research question. The purpose of the research and the problem for the research are interrelated and require that a correlation be shown.

THE RESEARCH HYPOTHESIS

The research hypothesis is a statement of the relationship of the variables that is anticipated by the researcher. Variables are characteristics, properties, traits, or personal attributes observed in a study that vary or possess different values. Examples of variables are ages, weights, or symptoms. The hypothesis is a declarative statement of a prediction or a hunch and follows the research question(s). It is frequently thought of as the researcher's educated or calculated guess as to the study question's answer(s). The hypothesis may consist of one or more statements of prediction that are directly derived from the research question. Examples of hypotheses derived from research questions are shown in Table 3–2.

Frequently novice researchers spend days in an attempt to formulate an appropriate hypothesis when the research problem denotes an inductive research question that does not require one. The way in which the research question is formulated, as discussed in Chapter 1, will indicate to the researcher the need for a hypothesis. Once the research question has been refined and assessed using the previously discussed criteria for well-developed researchable questions, the hypothesis is transposed from the question form of the research question to a statement form that is usually preceded by the words, *there will be* . . . . The hypothesis is always reported as being either supported or rejected.

Some research studies state the hypothesis in a null or statistical form. The null hypothesis reflects a statement in which the prediction suggests there is no significant statistical relationship of the variables.

THE CONCEPTUAL FRAMEWORK

The conceptual framework is an inherent step in the research process and may be viewed as an umbrellalike structure that encompasses the major ideas or concepts indicated by the research question. Developed through a logical and rationally written format, the conceptual framework explains, describes, and analyzes these ideas or concepts in order to provide the rationale for the proposed research.[14] The conceptual framework essentially provides an overview of what is currently known about the research question by focusing upon existing theories, completed research studies, related assumptions, and philosophical beliefs.[15] The conceptual framework is frequently viewed as the essential *link* between the research question and the appropriate methodological approach.

Beginning researchers are frequently confused by the requirements dictated by the review of the literature and the conceptual framework. The review of the literature is concerned with current information about the general problem proposed by the

TABLE 3–2

Research question:
    Does the introduction of a patient's medication handout increase the incidence of compliance with prescribed medication regimens by outpatient clients at a veterans' hospital?

Hypothesis:
    There will be a greater percentage of compliance with prescribed medication regimens by outpatient clients who receive a patient medication handout than by those outpatient clients who do not receive the patient medication handout at a veterans' hospital.

Research question:
    Does the introduction of a "pill ring" influence the patients' compliance with a prescribed seizure medication regimen as evidenced by therapeutic anticonvulsant blood levels?

Hypothesis:
    The introduction of a "pill ring" will increase patients' compliance with a prescribed seizure medication regimen as evidenced by their therapeutic anticonvulsant blood levels.

Research question:
    What are the perceptions of a Panel Selection Process for hospital staff positions as viewed by the panel members and the prospective candidates?

Hypothesis:
    Not needed, as the research question reflects an exploratory field study.

Research question:
    Is there a higher incidence of phlebitis in patients in Intensive Care Units who have intravenous care performed by the nurse every 48 hours than in those patients whose intravenous care is performed by the nurse every 24 hours?

Hypothesis:
    There will be no difference in the incidence of phlebitis in those patients who have intravenous care performed by the nurse every 48 hours than in those patients whose intravenous care is performed by the nurse every 24 hours. (null hypothesis)

research.[16] The conceptual framework, in contrast, involves an in-depth exploration of the concepts indicated by the conceptualized research question.[17,18] Beginning nurse researchers are also confused by the difference between the terms *conceptual framework* and *theoretical framework*. Although these terms are frequently used interchangeably by different authors, they are not the same. The conceptual framework is a more loosely conceived and broadly based organization of two or more concepts that are related to a common theme.[19,20] The theoretical framework, in contrast, is composed of formulated deductive propositions that state a particular relationship exists between the concepts.[21] The theoretical framework represents a higher level of development, as formulations between and among the identified concepts are able to predict and explain phenomena. Conceptual frameworks, although developed on a lower level than the theoretical framework, are viewed as precursors to the generation of theory.[22]

SUMMARY

The purpose of this chapter was twofold: (1) to identify the significance of the research question and discuss the development of researchable problems/questions, and (2) to describe the research purpose, the hypothesis, and the conceptual framework of the research process. The process of developing researchable problems and transposing them to research questions requires the transposition of the problem statement to a question. Discovery of researchable problems requires the sensitizing of oneself to everyday thoughts, observations, and experiences. Cues to our thoughts, observations, and experiences are manifested through verbalized or nonverbalized expressions of a *gripe,* a *wish,* a *bolt of lightning,* a *question,* a *challenge,* or *extrasensory perception.* Readings and theories, in addition, offer ideas for researchable problems.

Researchable problems, once formulated and developed into the research question, can be assessed for their quality on the basis of five criteria. The five criteria include clarity, significance, testing feasibility, measurability, and the relationship of the variables. Research questions that suggest a yes-no answer, a should-could connotation, or an opinion are poor research questions.

The purpose of the research process reflects the *why* of the research being proposed. The hypothesis is a hunch or a prediction about the research being proposed and follows the research question in the research proposal process. The hypothesis is stated as a definitive prediction, beginning with the words, *there will be.* The conceptual framework is an umbrellalike structure that encompasses the major ideas or concepts specifically indicated by the research question. It provides a link between the research question and the methodological approach.

QUESTIONS FOR STUDY AND DISCUSSION

1 Explain the significance of the research question to the inherent steps in the research process.

2 Describe three major areas from which researchable problems may be conceived.

3 Discuss three cues to developing researchable problems.

4 Explain the statement, "Each identified researchable problem will represent the individual's own uniqueness."

5 Compare and contrast the research problem and the research question.

6 Describe the value of using nursing theory as a basis for developing researchable problems.

7 Name the five stated criteria for assessing researchable problems.

8 Explain why the criteria of measurability and a relationship of the variables cannot always be achieved.

9 Given the three barriers, or stoppers, to well-developed researchable questions, develop in writing an example of each.

10 Differentiate the research purpose and the research problem.

11 Define the research hypothesis.

12 Based on a current area of interest, formulate in writing a researchable problem.

13 Explain the purpose of the conceptual framework.

REFERENCES

1 Pamela J. Brink, and Marilyn J. Wood, *Basic Steps in Planning Research from Question to Proposal,* 2d ed., Wadsworth Health Sciences Division, Belmont, California, 1983, p. 5.

2 Marjorie Batey, "Conceptualizing the Research Process," *Nursing Research,* vol. 20, no. 4, 1971, pp. 296–301.

3 Marjorie Batey, "Problem Identification and the Research Design," *Communicating Nursing Research,* Western Interstate Commission for Higher Education, Boulder, Colorado, October, 1969, p. 6.

4 Patricia A. Dempsey and Arthur D. Dempsey, *The Research Process in Nursing,* Van Nostrand, New York, 1981, p. 35.

5 Donna Diers, "Finding Clinical Problems for Study," *Journal of Nursing Administration,* November–December, 1971, vol. 1, no. 6, pp. 15–18.

6 Batey, op. cit., "Conceptualizing the Research Process," pp. 296–301.

7 Fred Kerlinger, *Foundations of Behavioral Research,* 2d ed., Holt, Rinehart, and Winston, New York, 1973, p. 3.

8 Kerlinger, ibid., p. 18.

9 Kerlinger, ibid., p. 17.

10 Florence S. Downs, *A Source Book of Nursing Research,* 3d ed., Davis, Philadelphia, 1984, p. 2.

11 Eleanor W. Treece, and James W. Treece, Jr., *Elements in Research in Nursing,* 3d ed., Mosby, St. Louis, 1982, p. 65.

12 Lucille E. Notter, *Essentials of Nursing Research,* Springer, New York, 1974, p. 38.

13 Denise Polit, and Bernadette Hungler, *Nursing Research: Principles and Methods,* 2d ed., Lippincott, Philadelphia, 1983, p. 71.

14 Brink and Wood, op. cit., pp. 44–46.

15 Donna Diers, *Research in Nursing Practice,* Lippincott, Philadelphia, 1979, p. 106.

16 Mary Ann Sweeney, and Peter Olivieri, *An Introduction to Nursing Research,* Lippincott, Philadelphia, 1981, pp. 93–94.

17 Brink and Wood, op. cit., pp. 44–46.

18 Sweeney and Olivieri, loc. cit.

19 Sydney D. Krampitz, and Natalie Pavlovich, *Readings for Nursing Research,* Mosby, St. Louis, 1981, p. 17.

20 Polit and Hungler, op. cit. p. 104.

21 Polit and Hungler, op. cit. p. 115.

22 Krampitz and Pavlovich, loc. cit.

BIBLIOGRAPHY

Brink, Pamela J., and Marilyn J. Wood. *Basic Steps in Planning Nursing Research from Question to Proposal,* 2d ed., Wadsworth Health Sciences Division, Belmont, California, 1983.

Dempsey, Patricia Ann, and Arthur D. Dempsey, *The Research Process in Nursing,* Van Nostrand, New York, 1981.

Diers, Donna: *Research in Nursing Practice,* Lippincott, Philadelphia, 1979.

Fleming, Juanita W., "Selecting a Clinical Nursing Problem for Research," *Image: The Journal of Nursing Scholarship,* vol. 16, no. 2, 1984, pp. 62–64.

Fox, David J: *Fundamentals of Research in Nursing,* 4th ed., Appleton-Century-Crofts, New York, 1982.

Fuller, Ellen: "Selecting a Clinical Problem for Research," *Image: The Journal of Nursing Scholarship,* vol. 14, no. 2, 1982, pp. 60–61.

Krampitz, Sydney D., and Natalie Pavlovich: *Readings for Nursing Research,* Mosby, St. Louis, 1981.

Lindeman, Carol W., and Donna Schantz: "The Research Question," *The Journal of Nursing Administration,* vol. 12, no., 1, 1982, pp. 6–10.

Polit, Denise, and Bernadette Hungler: *Nursing Research: Principles and Methods,* 2d ed., Lippincott, Philadelphia, 1983.

Sweeney, Mary Ann, and Peter Olivieri: *An Introduction to Nursing Research,* Lippincott, Philadelphia, 1981.

Verhonick, Phyllis J., and Catherine C. Seamon: *Research Methods for Undergraduate Students in Nursing,* Appleton-Century-Crofts, New York, 1978.

CHAPTER 4

THE LITERATURE REVIEW

Once a problem for study has been tentatively identified, the researcher will begin a thorough and systematic review of the literature. As the literature review progresses, the tentative problem may be refined, revised considerably, or changed completely if the researcher decides, based on the findings in the literature, that the problem already has been studied extensively by others or that the problem is not worth extensive study. More often, however, the literature review will confirm that the tentative problem previously identified is a major problem that needs investigation.

A researchable problem may first be determined *after* a review of literature in a specific field. However, the *best* problems for research usually emerge from the researcher's own hunches, ideas, beliefs, and nursing experiences. If one has to *look* and *search* for a problem to study, personal involvement, interest, and commitment are often less intense and ongoing than if the problem were one that has personally been felt as an irritation or "rock in the shoe" of the researcher.

PURPOSES OF THE LITERATURE REVIEW

There are several major purposes of the literature review. The most important of these are to:

- Identify, clarify, and/or refine a researchable problem.
- Strengthen the rationale and purpose of the research.
- Select an appropriate theoretical/conceptual framework for the study.
- Adapt methodological approaches utilized in other types of studies.
- Consider recommendations made in other similar types of studies.

Identify, Clarify, and/or Refine the Problem

The process of problem identification and statement is presented in Chapter 3. When one is reading a specific textbook, journal article, or other reference, ideas for problems often emerge. Inquisitive nurses, for example, will find themselves asking "why" after reading a particular fact or statement. Or, perhaps the reader is looking for more content or rationale when a paragraph or sentence seems to end abruptly without answering the questions in the reader's mind. The nurse is encouraged to make notes of or place question marks in the margin of the page when this occurs. Some of these questions could develop into researchable problems. Many journal articles and a few textbooks will state that further research is needed in a particular area when specific content is being discussed. The nurse researcher should be alert for such comments because they often lead to the formation of researchable problems.

Ideally, a tentatively identified problem becomes more clear as the literature review progresses. The refinement of the problem statement and the literature review occur almost simultaneously. The literature review broadens the reader's perspective, which ironically can help to state the problem more clearly because of a greater understanding of the problem. The more one reads about a particular topic, the more one is able to understand the total problem and thus succinctly write the problem statement and research questions.

Strengthen the Rationale and Purpose of the Research

Another major purpose of the literature review is to demonstrate that there is a need for study of the problem. As the researcher reads more and more about a particular problem, he or she becomes firmly convinced that the problem is a real one because a number of authors have stated that the problem occurs in various settings. On the other hand, the researcher may find that the problem has been studied extensively and that results and several possible solutions are already available. At other times, there may be very little, if any, literature published relating to the problem. This situation could mean that no one has recognized the problem or that there has been nothing published on the topic. When the researcher can find nothing in the literature on a topic of interest, as may very well happen in some areas of nursing, the lack does not mean that the problem is not worth studying. In fact, a lack of available literature on a specific topic may strengthen the need for study of the topic because it may indicate that no one else has identified or studied the problem.

Select an Appropriate Theoretical/Conceptual Framework for the Study

As discussed in Chapters 1 and 2, extensive research in a particular area may lead a researcher to formulate a specific theory that is aimed to serve as a basis for nursing practice. This type of research is currently being conducted by nurse scholars and researchers at the postdoctoral level. Beginning nurse researchers, however, will want to find theoretical or conceptual frameworks upon which to build their studies. In the past, as noted in Chapter 2, nurse researchers primarily utilized theories or concepts from fields other than nursing as a framework for their studies. Now nurses are utilizing nursing theories as frameworks for their research. Only when these theories are tested again and again in various settings will they be shown to have a major role in nursing practice.

Adapt Methodological Approaches Used by Others

While reading studies conducted by experienced nurse researchers, the beginning nurse researcher will start to become familiar with a variety of methodological approaches and research designs. While the approach and design to be used must be appropriate for the problem, ideas for methodology can be studied and possibly adapted for use with a similar research problem. The nurse is encouraged to read as many research articles as possible in the major nursing research journals. The more research reports read, the more familiar the nurse will become with the total research process.

Consider Recommendations Made in Other Similar Types of Studies

One of the concerns in nursing research is the fact that there has been limited replication (repetition) of studies. Because a particular problem has been studied one or more times is no reason that the same problem should not be studied again. Once most researchers have completed a study and written a report, they recognize that there are many aspects of the study that they should have done differently that could have strengthened or influenced their results in one way or another.

Results of a study can only be generalized to the population from which the sample came. Therefore, a similar study could be conducted utilizing recommendations made by previous researchers in published articles (such as sample size or control of specific variables). Or, exactly the same study could be carried out with a different population in a different setting or geographical location in an attempt to determine if the results would be the same. If such is the case, however, the researcher will need to obtain written permission from the author and/or publisher to utilize the design and instruments, if applicable. Most researchers encourage (and in fact are often quite pleased by) requests to replicate their studies.

SOURCES FOR THE SEARCH

The library is an essential tool of the researcher. The nurse will find that the library holds the key to research endeavors. One of the first goals of the beginning researcher should be to become completely oriented to a specific library setting. If the library to be used does not provide for a specific orientation for new users, nurses should seek an orientation for themselves. One of the reference librarians is usually the person to ask about a tour or orientation. The librarian will be glad to provide for an orientation and/or assist with specific questions that may occur later.

Nursing Resources

The nurse researcher should begin the literature review by searching and utilizing the major nursing resources in the library. Specific sources that will be discussed here are listed below:

1 Nursing indexes
  a *Cumulative Index to Nursing and Allied Health Literature*
  b *Nursing Studies Index*
  c *International Nursing Index*
2 Nursing journals
3 Nursing books
4 Dissertation abstracts/listings

Nursing Indexes.   Before using any index for the first time, the reader should become thoroughly familiar with what the index includes and how to use it. Checking the directions and outline of contents at the beginning of any volume will facilitate the use of the index by the reader. There are three major indexes to nursing literature.

Cumulative Index to Nursing and Allied Health Literature   The *Cumulative Index to Nursing Literature* was the first nursing index to be published (in 1961) and covers the years from 1956 to the present. It is the only index for the years 1960 to 1965. The name was changed to *Cumulative Index to Nursing and Allied Health Literature* (CINAHL) in 1977. It is published bimonthly by Glendale Adventist Medical Center Publications Service, Glendale, California, and issues are combined into an annual cumulation. The Index is currently organized into a subject section, author section, and appendix (audiovisual materials, book reviews, and pamphlets).[1]

The CINAHL is probably the most useful of the three nursing indexes because it is ongoing and includes the most recent references in nursing. Another advantage is that the Index labels research-related articles with a letter R, which will help the nurse to find research references more quickly.

Nursing Studies Index.   The *Nursing Studies Index* (NSI) is the "only comprehensive historical survey of research in nursing as published during the first sixty years of this century."[2] It lists analytical, historical, and biographical nursing literature from the years 1900 to 1959, and it is the only index to nursing literature for the years 1900 to 1956. For this reason, it is an excellent general source of references for historical research.

The NSI is composed of four volumes, as shown in Table 4–1. It is the only nursing index that has annotated references (a brief discussion of the author and summary of the content). The NSI includes a subject, author, and agency or organization index.

International Nursing Index.   The *International Nursing Index* (INI) is sponsored by the American Nurses' Association and it is published quarterly by the American

TABLE 4–1
THE NURSING STUDIES INDEX[2]

Volume	Covers Years	Date of Publication
I	1900–1929	1972
II	1930–1949	1970
III	1950–1956	1966
IV	1957–1959	1963

Journal of Nursing Company in cooperation with the National Library of Medicine. The INI contains references to articles in over 200 nursing journals from all over the world for the years 1966 to the present. It also includes references to many nonnursing journals and journals printed in other than the English language.[3] The researcher may not find this index as useful as the other two because many of the journals listed will not be available in the local library. However, if a journal article is found that is particularly pertinent to the topic being studied and there is a dearth of such references, the library can be requested to search for the journal in another library and obtain a copy of the specific article for the researcher. There is a list of doctoral dissertations in the annual index, which gives an additional source of recent research topics that may be helpful.

Nursing Journals. The number of published nursing journals has been increasing tremendously in the past few years. The first nursing journal was the *American Journal of Nursing,* which was first published on October 1, 1900[4] and has been published continuously ever since. The nurse who is interested in historical research or any nurse who explores some of those early issues will find the content interesting. *Nursing Research* was first published in 1952 and *Nursing Outlook* in 1953.[5] As specialization developed in nursing, many new and specialized nursing journals have been published. There are now over 100 nursing and nursing-related journals and new ones are published every year.[6] Appendix A lists sample nursing journals with the publisher, address, and primary focus of each one. No attempt has been made to present a complete list. However, the researcher may find this information useful to decide which if any of the journals are to be reviewed and/or purchased for individual use.

While many of these journals publish the results of research studies occasionally, there are only a few whose primary goal is to publish and disseminate research findings. The journals that are primarily devoted to research are listed below. More information on each of these journals will be found in Appendix A.

Advances in Nursing Science
Nursing Research
Nursing Research Report
Research in Nursing and Health
Western Journal of Nursing Research

The *refereed* journal is considered by many to "bring higher prestige to authors appearing in them than nonrefereed journals do,"[7] although the definition of what refereed means is less clear.[8] A refereed journal is generally considered to be "one which utilizes a system of prepublication review by three or more readers, selected because of their expertise, who judge the merit of manuscripts according to criteria established by the journal."[9] These reviews are blind; the reviewers do not know the author's name and the author does not know who has reviewed the manuscript. This process of peer review is supposed to be more objective and result in the publication of higher-quality articles.[10]

The nurse should become familiar with as many of the nursing journals as possible. At the least, the nurse should regularly review one of the major research journals for studies of interest as well as one or more journals in the major field of interest and/or specialization.

Nursing Books.   Although most current research is published in the nursing journals, there are some classic ongoing studies that have been published in books; for example, *Reality Shock* by Marlene Kramer.[11] The nurse researcher must not overlook this source. Resources for such references will be found in the library catalogue or through computer searches (discussed later in the chapter).

A *Guide to Library Resources for Nursing* by Strauch and Brundage[12] may assist the nurse to learn more about nursing as well as general resources in the library. This book also includes an annotated bibliography of major books and journals in nursing, which are categorized according to numerous clinical specialty areas as well as many related fields, such as pharmacology, nutrition, and anatomy and physiology. There is also a specific section on references related to research, grants, and statistics.

Other nursing books that will be helpful to the nurse researcher:

• *Annual Review of Nursing Research* (Volume 1 was edited by Harriett H. Werley and Joyce J. Fitzpatrick and was published by the Springer Publishing Company in 1983. The book includes contributed reviews of nursing research on a variety of topics related to nursing practice, nursing care delivery, and the profession of nursing.)

• *Facts About Nursing* (This includes current statistics on registered nurses and related professions and facilities, and it is published periodically by the American Nurses' Association.)

Dissertation Abstracts/Listings.   There are several sources of dissertation abstracts and listings of recent doctoral dissertations. An abstract is a *secondary* source that gives the specific bibliographical data for a reference as well as a very short description of the article and/or research study. The researcher can decide from the brief description if the *primary* source (where the study was first published) should be read for details and critique.

Besides the INI previously mentioned, other nursing sources give abstracts or listings of dissertations recently completed. Some of these are:

• *Reflections* (official newsletter of Sigma Theta Tau, national nursing honor society, which lists titles of recent doctoral dissertations completed by its members)

• American Nurses' Foundation *Bulletin* (includes abstracts of studies by nurses that have been funded by the American Nurses' Foundation)

• *Directory of Nurses with Doctoral Degrees 1984* (published by the American Nurses' Association, Inc., and includes current research activities of nurses listed)

If the researcher's address is not given in these publications, the name of the school where the dissertation was completed is usually listed, so that the researcher can be contacted for more information. Reviewing abstracts of recently completed doctoral dissertations and/or other current research in nursing can give the novice researcher many excellent ideas about topics being studied in nursing. Often researchers will find that others have just completed studies on topics that they are also interested in pursuing.

If more information is needed than that available in the abstract, the nurse can request that the library obtain a copy of the entire dissertation or a microfilm of the dissertation through interlibrary loan.

In addition, there is an annual publication in the library, *Comprehensive Dissertation Index*, which includes nursing dissertations in the Sciences, Part I, Health Sciences section. There is also an annual Author Index, which may be helpful if the researcher is interested in finding an abstract of a dissertation completed by a specific nurse researcher. Once the author's name has been found in the Index, the dissertation abstract can be found in the appropriate volume of *Dissertation Abstracts International Section B Sciences and Engineering*.

Related Library Resources

Although the nurse researcher will primarily utilize nursing literature, the review of literature should not be limited to nursing references. Related library resources that the nurse may want to investigate are listed below:

- *Abridged Index Medicus*
- Biological and psychological abstracts
- *Reader's Guide*
- Computer searches

Abridged Index Medicus. The *Index Medicus* is the comprehensive medical index to periodicals collected by the National Library of Medicine. It is the most complete source for biomedical research and could be consulted *after* using the nursing indexes. References on recent medical research that may influence nursing research and/or practice will be found in the *Abridged Index Medicus*. References cited in the *New England Journal of Medicine*, one of the oldest and most respected medical journals, for example, often include recent research findings that have implications for nursing. The *Abridged Index Medicus* is usually found in the reference department of the library.

Biological and Psychological Abstracts. The biological and psychological abstracts are possible sources of research findings that may be helpful in clarifying a particular nursing problem. Each of these are separate publications that briefly describe current publications and research studies in these particular fields. The fields of biology and psychology often assist in the formulation and/or clarification of a conceptual or theoretical framework for the nursing problem to be studied.

Reader's Guide. The Reader's Guide is a basic index to periodical literature that is primarily in popular magazines rather than professional literature. However, sometimes the nurse will want to read lay references that are related to a particular topic for information or interest. Examples of popular magazines that may have current articles related to health care are *Time, Today's Health*, and *Modern Maturity*. The nurse should recognize, however, that these resources do not contain research articles and that they would not be acceptable as references in the review of the literature for a research study.

Computer Searches. The use of computer searches has decreased dramatically the time needed for the review of literature in the research process. Most university and college libraries have the capability for computer data base literature searching. The researcher should seek assistance from the reference librarian to learn how and where to request this search.

One of the librarians in the reference department will be able to help the researcher determine what types of literature should be searched. That is, depending on the topic of the research, the search will focus primarily on biological, sociological, or medical literature. Examples of the major types of computer data bases of interest to nurses are:

- Nursing and Allied Health Literature Index (This data base was initiated in 1984 and is the first online data base specifically for nursing and allied health. It is produced by the *Cumulative Index to Nursing and Allied Health Literature* and begins with records from January, 1983)
- MEDLARS (Medical Literature Analysis and Retrieval System)
- MEDLINE (Medlars on Line is a major source for biomedical literature and is produced by the United States National Library of Medicine)
- ERIC (educational materials from the Educational Resources Information Center)
- Critical Care Medical Library (references in the fields of emergency and critical care medicine)
- Drug Information Fulltext (information on the stability, chemistry, pharmacokinetics, action, usage, dosage, and administration of more than 1000 drugs)
- International Pharmaceutical Abstracts (information on the development and use of drugs from the clinical, practical, theoretical, economic, and scientific aspects)
- Embase (biomedical journals; topics included are environmental health, pollution control, forensic science, health economics, hospital management, and public health)
- Cancerlit (includes a wide variety of published and unpublished materials from medicine, nursing, the biological sciences, philosophy, religion, law, and the behavioral sciences; sponsored by the National Cancer Institute and contains more than 300,000 references relating to cancer)
- Popline (references on topics such as family planning, fertility control, population, and reproduction)
- Health Planning and Administration (includes nonclinical references on health planning and administration, health insurance, quality assurance, licensing, accreditation, and health care delivery.

The data base services librarian will need to determine from the researcher key words related to the research problem. It is important to limit these words to those that are most directly related to the topic of the research study. For example, if the study involves teaching newly diagnosed diabetics who are adolescents how to give themselves insulin, the researcher would need to use many more key words than *diabetes*. If only the word *diabetes* were used, thousands of references would be found by the computer. Not only would the references be too general to be helpful, but if the researcher has to pay for computer time and the print out of listings, it would be quite expensive.

Instead, key words to use might be *diabetes, adolescents,* and *insulin.* Even then, there would probably be a large number of references, so the computer search should be limited and as closely related to the research problem as possible.

A decision will also need to be made about how many years back the literature should be searched. Unless the research is of an historical nature, three to five years is usually considered adequate.

The researcher usually has a choice of requesting (1) a print out with an alphabetical list of references, or (2) a print out with an alphabetical list of annotated references. The researcher will make a careful review of the list to determine which of the references will be read for a closer analysis and possible use in the literature review.

General Library Resources

Some of the *general* library sources that may be helpful to the nurse researcher are the:

Library Catalogue
United States Government publications
Interlibrary loan

Library Catalogue.   The primary tool for finding books in a library is its catalogue. Until recently most libraries maintained a card catalogue, so-called because it was an extensive alphabetical index consisting of 3 × 5 cards. Every book in the library is generally represented in the index by cards filed for the author(s) of the book, for the title of the book, and for each of several subjects in the book. This system enables researchers to discover the book by a variety of means, but it does require accurate knowledge of at least one of the following: the correctly spelled full name of the author(s), the correct title, or one's subject of interest expressed in correct Library of Congress vocabulary.

Now, many libraries are converting the card index to machine readable form, and, as part of progress in that direction, some have produced their catalogue on microfiche (a sheet of transparent film holding multiple pages) or microfilm (long strip of 16mm or 35mm film). Eventually, most libraries expect to have an outline computer catalogue. No matter what format is used by the academic library, it is necessary to seek careful instruction in its use. The researcher should assume nothing until having been given an adequate demonstration in the use of the library catalogue and should seek assistance from the library staff when problems or questions arise.

Careful searching of the information contained in the catalogue will enable a researcher to choose intelligently from among possible books before visiting the book stacks. One can, for example, eliminate books too old to be of reliable value by their publication dates or identify books with tables and maps. This type of information is in all standard catalogue formats.

United States government publications.   Numerous government publications are available on a variety of topics related to health care and nursing. Examples of federal publications are those prepared by: (1) Centers for Disease Control (CDC); (2) Federal Drug Administration (FDA); (3) Department of Health and Human Services (DHHS);

(4) Health Services Administration (HSA); (5) National Institute of Health (NIH); (6) National Institute of Mental Health (NIMH); and (7) Public Health Service. Some of the periodicals prepared by these agencies will be available in the periodicals section or the reference department of the library. Many government documents are not listed in the library catalogue, although the library may have them. The reference librarian should be consulted for available documents. A *Monthly Catalogue of United States Government Publications* lists all publications issued during a given month by all government agencies. Specific publications not available in the library may be ordered from the following source:

Superintendent of Documents
U.S. Government Printing Office
Washington, D.C. 20402

Usually there is no fee for these publications if ordered in single copies.

A specific example of a United States government publication is census data records. The census has been taken every ten years in the United States since 1790.[13] If specific population data about a particular state, county, city, or census tract within a city is needed to determine possible population groups for study, for example, the most recent census data may be helpful. Census data are found in the reference department of most large libraries.

Interlibrary loan.   If a needed book cannot be found in the library catalogue, the book will not be in the library. If a specific book is needed and it is not available, the book may be ordered through interlibrary loan. The exact author, title, edition, and date is needed so that the librarian may request the book from another nearby library. Master's theses and doctoral dissertations in nursing that have been completed in a university with a graduate program, for example, may be obtained through interlibrary loan by students who need to read these primary sources for research on a particular topic. Many universities provide this service only for faculty and graduate students, however, so the researcher should consult with the librarian. Also, the process may take one to several weeks, depending upon a number of variables in the process, and a fee may be required. Some universities place their dissertations on microfilm and copies of these may be purchased.

GENERAL FACTORS TO CONSIDER IN THE SELECTION OF LITERATURE

While the library search of all references related to the research problem or questions proceeds, the researcher will choose the ones to be used in the literature review. Some of the factors to be considered in making this selection are:

- Date of references
- Quality of references
- Primary versus secondary sources
- Use of nursing-related and general references
- Number of references

Date of References

The most current resources should be used, usually those published in the last five years. Most books and many periodicals report on studies that were conducted at least one to two years before the publication date because that is usually how long it takes to write the report and have it published. Thus, a book published five years ago might include research findings of seven or more years earlier. For this reason, dissertation abstracts in journals may provide more current research results.

If the research is historical, however, all references pertinent to the topic of study, both old and new, may be used. *Classic* studies related to a research problem should also be used, even if they are old. These are usually studies that are well known on a particular topic, such as the Framingham study on risk factors in heart disease. If more recent research refutes previous conclusions, however, the researcher must be aware of these studies and use them in the literature review.

Quality of References

The references used in the literature review should be of high quality. The journal in which the study is published should be evaluated. If the journal is a well-established one that is refereed and has a wide circulation and a good reputation among the readers for whom it is intended, it will more than likely have high-quality articles.

The names of nurses on the editorial review board should also help the reader to evaluate the quality of the articles in the journal. If the reviewers are well-known nursing leaders who have written high-quality books or articles, it is likely that the articles published in a specific journal have been chosen because of their quality. The reader should refer to Chapter 8 for more details in learning how to read and evaluate specific research articles.

Primary versus Secondary Sources

It is very important that the researcher utilize primary rather than secondary resources in the literature review. *Primary resources* refer to the original article or published report of a study by the researcher who conducted the study. Parts of the study, for example the methodology or conclusions, will often be referred to in the review of literature in later studies written by different authors. However, the second author may be stating his or her own interpretation of the original study, thus allowing for some distortion of the methodology or results.

Some research abstracts are also written by someone other than the original researcher. Research abstracts tend to be very concise and are therefore not appropriate as a literature source. The abstract is meant to help the researcher evaluate the topic of the research and determine if the original study should be read. These reviews and abstracts are types of *secondary sources,* which are not appropriate in a literature review. It is often frustrating to the researcher when the original resource is not readily available in the library. If such is the case, the researcher should seek assistance from one of the librarians to determine how to locate the original source. Perhaps a nearby medical school or hospital library will have the primary source needed. Or if there is time, interlibrary loan may be used.

Use of Nursing-Related and General References

Although the literature review should focus on studies and articles found in the nursing literature, nurse researchers should not limit themselves to such literature. The literature review may be strengthened and enhanced by the use of theories, concepts, principles, and research findings from other types of related literature. For example, literature in sociology and/or anthropology may be needed to help explain a phenomenon or problem in a study of how elderly Hispanics evaluate the health care delivery system in the United States. Studies of management and organizational behavior in the field of business may give clues about how to study the head nurse's role or work satisfaction among nurses in a general hospital.

Number of References

As discussed later in Chapter 9, the research proposal will contain only selected references, but a sufficient number are needed to help provide a rationale for the study. The final research report will contain all relevant and important references, including those utilized in the research proposal.

When the researcher begins to experience the circular syndrome; that is, begins to see the same or similar findings in many studies, or when many of the references at the end of an article are those that have already been reviewed, this is usually an indication that the major studies/references related to the problem have been found. The most recent journals, however, also need to be reviewed for relevant studies as they are published so that the review will be as up to date as possible.

While the researcher is expected to have a comprehensive review of the most recent related literature, the quality of the study is not determined by the length of the list of references. One should not attempt to "pad" the bibliography with duplicated or irrelevant references. A summary of the factors to be considered in making the literature selection will be found in Table 4–2.

TABLE 4–2
FACTORS TO BE CONSIDERED IN MAKING THE LITERATURE SELECTION

1. Use references published within the last five years.
2. Choose references from nursing journals that are considered to be of high quality.
3. Use primary resources rather than secondary sources.
4. Include references from other than nursing journals where appropriate.
5. Refrain from padding the literature review with unrelated or minimally related articles just to have an extensive bibliography.
6. When there are many articles that have the same or similar content, include only the one or two most relevant.
7. Review the reference list and bibliography at the end of articles read to determine if some of the items listed would be pertinent to the study.
8. Rarely, if ever, utilize references from lay magazines unless it is to make a particular point specifically related to the research.

ORGANIZING THE LITERATURE FINDINGS

The researcher should learn to use an organized and systematic method of collecting, recording, and storing the results of the literature search. For example, one should choose and be consistent in the use of an accepted bibliographical format (see Chapter 9). When taking initial notes from a reference, the exact bibliographical format should be used that will be used in the research proposal and the final report to prevent confusion and save time when preparing the written reports.

All of the bibliographical data for each reference should be collected and recorded at the time the reference is read and summarized. Having to look up a reference more than one time because the exact title was not recorded correctly or because the volume of the journal or the inclusive page numbers are missing is a waste of valuable time.

If a specific short quote is essential, it should be written exactly as is it appears, within quotation marks; the page number where the quote can be found should be recorded so that it can be used in the list of references.

The method of organizing and storing the reference information will vary, but *some specific method should be used consistently*. A loose-leaf notebook, a spiral notebook, or 5 × 8 lined cards may be chosen. A sample of the latter may be found in Figure 4–1. This sample gives the general topic, date read, complete bibliographical data, and the essential points (not necessarily complete sentences), with specific page numbers of pertinent content and specific quotes. A collection of such cards will assist researchers greatly when they begin to write the literature review for the research proposal and/or research report.

FIGURE 4–1
One suggested format for collecting and storing reference summaries.

DATE: 3/3/85	TOPIC: Family, home care
Hildebrandt, Eugenie D., "Respite Care in the Home, "AJN,	
vol. 83, no. 10, 1983, pp. 1428-1431	
p. 1428	- few respite programs in the US
	-"no clear consensus on a model for respite care"
	-nurse practitioner assesses the home and makes a plan of care
	-respite worker stays in home to relieve caregiver 4-72 hours
p. 1430	-publicized respite program in community
	-some families embarrassed to ask for help
	-caregivers need nurture themselves in order to help family member
p. 1431	-82% of care given to families of elderly in one year
	-cost of respite care less than institutionalization
	-helps to maintain dependent people in the home

WRITING THE REVIEW OF THE LITERATURE

After the needed references have been found, read, summarized, and recorded, all of the information needs to be brought together in a final summary labeled "The Review of the Literature." This section generally follows the research problem/questions/hypotheses. The written review of the literature is not just a compilation of sentences or short paragraphs from the various relevant references read. Instead, the literature review is organized in a logical and readable format that flows from broad background data of the problem to relevant recent studies, if available. The major points to be considered in writing the summary of the literature review will be found in Table 4–3.

Since one of the purposes of the literature review is to identify, clarify, and refine the research problem, it is important to develop a sound rationale for the need of the study. The discussion of classic studies related to the problem should be included. If there are conflicting findings among studies, they should be compared and contrasted.

The discussion should begin with broad references related to the study and end with the most recent pertinent studies. The review can be organized around the variables to be studied and/or the theoretical or conceptual framework of the study. The flow should proceed so that by the end of the review, the reader perceives that the problem is one worthy of research investigation.

The researcher may be concerned because relatively few references (especially research studies) have been found which specifically relate to the research problem. If such is the case, the review can simply state that fact. Such a statement may add to the rationale or purpose of the study because the identified problem has not been studied extensively. The researcher needs to be careful to state, however, that no relevant studies were found and not that there are no studies on this topic. There may be studies, perhaps unpublished at that point in time, that are directly relevant to the problem.

SUMMARY

The review of the literature is perhaps not the most interesting and creative aspect of research for many, but it is an early and essential step. The literature review helps the researcher to identify, clarify, refine, and confirm the research problem/questions. The review is also important in selecting and relating the problem to a theoretical/conceptual framework.

TABLE 4–3
MAJOR POINTS IN WRITING THE SUMMARY OF THE LITERATURE REVIEW

1. Write in an organized, logical, and readable manner.
2. Organization should flow from broad background data to relevant recent studies.
3. Build up to a sound rationale for the need for the study.
4. Compare and contrast conflicting findings from the literature review.
5. Include references of sufficient breadth and depth without repeating similar research findings.

The researcher needs to be completely familiar with the resources available in the library: nursing, nursing related, and general. Some of the most important resources include the: (1) *Cumulative Index to Nursing and Allied Health Literature,* (2) *Nursing Studies Index,* (3) *International Nursing Index,* (4) nursing journals and books; (5) *Abridged Index Medicus;* (6) biological and psychological abstracts; (7) library catalogue; and (8) United States government publications. Computer data bases, such as the Nursing and Allied Health Literature Index, MEDLINE, and Cancerlit are excellent time-saving sources. The researcher should identify and utilize a systematic method of collecting and recording information from these sources to facilitate the written review and prevent wasting time in searching for a reference more than once.

The written literature review should be comprehensive, but not padded; utilize references within the last five years, unless you are doing historical research; contain breadth as well as depth; discuss conflicting findings; and be written in a clear, logical, and organized manner.

QUESTIONS FOR STUDY AND DISCUSSION

1 Discuss *two* purposes of the literature review.

2 How is the literature review related to the theoretical/conceptual framework for the study?

3 Name and describe the *three* major nursing indexes.

4 What are *three* nursing journals that publish nursing research?

5 What is the *Abridged Index Medicus* and where is it located in most libraries?

6 Name *two* general library sources that can be used in the literature search.

7 What are some general factors to consider in the selection of literature? (See Table 4–2.)

8 What factors should be considered in writing the review of the literature?

REFERENCES

1 Katina P. Strauch, and Dorothy J. Brundage, *Guide to Library Resources for Nursing,* Appleton-Century-Crofts, New York, 1980, pp. 16, 414.

2 *Nursing Studies Index,* filmstrip, The American Journal of Nursing Company, New York, 1976.

3 Strauch and Brundage, op. cit., pp. 17, 424.

4 Josephine A. Dolan, *Nursing in Society,* 13th ed., Saunders, Philadelphia, 1973, p. 254.

5 Dolan, op. cit., pp. 254–255.

6 Joanne Comi McCloskey, and Elizabeth Swanson, "Publishing Opportunities for Nurses: A Comparison of 100 Journals," *Image: The Journal of Nursing Scholarship,* vol. 14. no. 2, 1982, pp. 50–56.

7 Bonnie C. Clayton, and Kathleen Boyle, "The Refereed Journal: Prestige in Professional Publication," *Nursing Outlook,* vol. 29, no. 9, 1981, p. 531.

8 Lewis, Edith P., "A Peerless Publication" (editorial), *Nursing Outlook,* vol. 28, no. 4, 1980, p. 225.

9 Clayton and Boyle, op. cit., p. 534.

10 Clayton and Boyle, op. cit., p. 532.
11 Marlene Kramer, *Reality Shock,* Mosby, St. Louis, 1974.
12 Strauch and Brundage, op. cit.
13 Census Data, 1790–1890, National Archives and Records Service, General Services Administration, GSA-Wash DC 65–224.

BIBLIOGRAPHY

Sparks, Susan M., "The National Library of Medicine's Bibliographic Databases: Tools for Nursing Research," *Image: The Journal of Nursing Scholarship,* vol. 16, no. 1, 1984, pp. 24–27.

CHAPTER 5

METHODOLOGICAL APPROACHES TO RESEARCH

The way the research problem/question is conceptualized will dictate the most appropriate methodology used to conduct the proposed research. Methodological approaches to research refer to the broad areas of research that reflect the *factual* or *doing* activities inherent in the research process. The methodological approach provides the researcher the basic direction in answering the question: How can the research question be most appropriately answered or what path must be followed to obtain answers that are consistent with the question being asked?

In Chapter 1, three major categories of research, experimental, quasi-experimental, and field research studies (nonexperimental) were identified and placed on a research continuum. These three categories of research were developed according to a number of characteristics that included *how* the research question was conceptualized and *where* or in what setting the proposed research would be conducted. The *major categories* and their related characteristics provide the researcher with the basic direction in conducting research and, therefore, can be considered the broad *methodological approaches* to research. (The reader is encouraged to review Chapter 1, particularly the research continuum shown in Figure 1–1). *Types* of research, such as historical, descriptive, and exploratory, derive from the direction suggested by the broad methodological approaches and offer the researcher the most appropriate investigational mode to answer the research question (see Table 5–1). The research *design* is the detailed plan for implementing the research and encompasses the *specifics* of the research process, including the what, who, how, and when of the proposed research.[1]

The purpose of this chapter is to provide a foundation of research terminology, describe and differentiate the basic types of research, and identify the most commonly used research designs. The reader is encouraged to remember that some research questions conceptualized or developed in the clinical practice setting are not amenable to

TABLE 5–1
THE RESEARCH CONTINUUM
TYPES OF RESEARCH AND THEIR APPROXIMATE PLACEMENT*

Experimental	Quasi-experimental	Field Research Studies (Nonexperimental)
True experiment pretest posttest	Nonequivalent control group pretest posttest	Exploratory
		Hypothesis-testing
		Descriptive
		•Survey
		•Longitudinal Grounded theory
	Time Series	•Comparison
	Field experiment	•Correlational
		Ex post facto
		Case studies
		Historical

*Conceptualized problem dictates method and type of research with their respective designs

a specific research design.[2] The most appropriate research design may need to be developed by the researcher after decisions on implementation issues have been made.[3]

RESEARCH TERMINOLOGY

A profession may be characterized by a language its members use to communicate with each other. Nurse researchers not only use a language reflective of their profession but also terminology consistent with research. In order to understand the succeeding discussion of the types and accompanying designs of research, the following terms are presented. Additional research terms may be found in the glossary.

- *Variable.* The characteristic, property, trait, or attribute of a person that varies or takes on different values within the population under study. Variables represent concepts that are operationalized.
- *Independent variable.* The presumed cause, treatment given, and the manipulated or modified variable responsible for an effect.
- *Dependent variable.* The presumed effect caused from the introduction, modification, or manipulation of the treatment of the independent variable. The dependent variable may also be referred to as the *criterion measure.*
- *Extraneous variables.* Those variables that are not of direct interest to the researcher but could affect the variables being studied.
- *Intervening variable.* Variables in the experimental design that are thought to affect the relationship between the independent and dependent variable.

• *Sample*. A part or portion of the population that is believed to represent the characteristics of the population being considered for the study.

• *Hypothesis*. A positive declarative statement of the relationship between two or more variables; usually stated by the researcher as a prediction or a hunch and derived from the research question.

• *Instrument*. The tool by which the data are collected.

• *Data*. Plural for the word datum or the information being collected.

• *Validity*. The degree to which the instrument measures what it is supposed to measure.

• *Reliability*. The consistency or repeatability to which the instrument or tool connotes stability.

• *Pilot study*. A preliminary minisimulation of the proposed research.[4]

• *Definition of terms*. Principal terms of the research problem/question that the researcher has developed to denote particular meanings that may be different from the generally accepted meanings.

• *Quantitative research*. Research concerned with the quantification or measurement of data.

• *Qualitative research*. Research concerned with the collection, collation, and analysis of data that is not amenable to quantification.

• *Assumptions*. Basic principles of the proposed research that are accepted as being true on the basis of logic or reason without proof or verification.[5]

• *Limitations*. Weaknesses of the methods used, such as sampling procedures, uncontrolled variables, poor instrumentation, or compromises of internal and external validity, that may restrict the conclusions or generalizability of the findings.[6]

THE PILOT STUDY

Although the pilot study has been defined above, its importance to the success of the proposed research cannot be overemphasized. In many instances, the success or failure of the proposed research is dependent upon the results of the pilot study. The pilot study is a miniature version of the major research study and mimics or resembles the major research study in every detail. The pilot study thus incorporates all aspects of the research process from the identification of the research question to analysis of data and conclusions. The purpose of the pilot study is to provide the researcher an opportunity to implement the proposed research study on a *trial* basis. Pilot studies are conducted to: (1) determine the feasibility of the major study, (2) identify problems in the research design, (3) refine the data collection and analysis plan, (4) test the instrument to be used in the major study, and (5) provide the researcher some experience with the subject's methodology and instruments.[7] In addition, the pilot study provides the researcher an opportunity to become acquainted with the staff members of the clinical setting in which the research is to be conducted as well as to become familiar with the institutional policies and routines that guide the ongoing everyday activities. An understanding of the policies and routines of the institution will facilitate implementing the major research study without causing major disruptions in the delivery of health care activities to patients/clients.[8] Implementing the pilot study thus provides the researcher the opportunity to detect or discover any particular limitation that would cause problems or difficulties in conducting the major research study. Frequently, problems in relation to data collection concerning human subjects and reliability and validity issues as well as the control of variables are detected by conducting the pilot study.[9] Based on the outcome of the pilot study, adjustments or modifications to the proposed major research study can be made to ensure to a greater degree the success of the research.

The pilot study has limitations that must be considered by the researcher. Since the pilot study reflects a miniversion of the major research study, the problems or difficulties detected must be assessed accordingly by the researcher. Sometimes the problems that have been detected in the implementation of the pilot study reflect the small sample size, the limited scope of the study, or an unusual situation that occurred in the clinical setting. Although these problems warrant consideration by the researcher, they may or may not be sufficient reasons to adjust or modify the proposed research study.

Since the pilot study closely resembles the proposed major research, another limitation of the pilot study is the amount of time and effort required to conduct the pilot study. This limitation, however, can be alleviated by allowing sufficient time for the pilot study when the research time table or time schedule is initially developed.

The advantages of conducting a pilot study far outweigh the limitations. It is highly recommended that the beginning nurse researcher plan to conduct a pilot study in preparation for implementing and conducting the major research study. The pilot study offers the researcher the best means of identifying the strengths and weaknesses of the proposed research so improvements may be made and problems detected that must be resolved before the major study is attempted.[10]

TYPES OF RESEARCH

Based on the three major categories of research that represent the broad methodological approaches to research, several types of research may be derived. These types of research provide the researcher with a multiplicity of investigational modes by which researchable questions can be answered. To determine the type of research that is most appropriate, the research question must be assessed in relation to deductive or inductive thinking, the setting in which the research will be conducted, and the inherent characteristics of the three major categories of research discussed in Chapter 1. For the purposes of organization, the types of research will be discussed sequentially from those research questions that employ deductive thinking, use highly controlled settings, and seek quantitative data to those research questions that are conceived by inductive thinking, use loosely controlled settings, and seek qualitative data. The presentation of the types of research will, thus, approximate the research continuum (see Figure 1–1). The discussion of each type of research will include the purpose, characteristics, and strengths and weaknesses.

Experimental Research

Experimental type of research is the most scientific of all research approaches. According to Kerlinger, experimental research is the only true research approach.[11] Experimental research provides the rigid control of relevant variables that may be responsible for variance.[12] The purpose of experimental research is to investigate cause and effect relationships by exposing one or more treatment conditions and comparing the results to one or more control groups that did not receive the treatment.[13] In experimental research the researcher is an active agent in the experiment. The researcher manipulates and controls the treatment or independent variables and observes and measures the resulting variation on the dependent variable.

The experimental type of research is characterized by three criteria: *manipulation, control,* and *randomization.*[14] *Manipulation* refers to the active role the researcher plays in the experiment. The researcher introduces an independent variable by administering a selected treatment to the subjects of one or more groups (experimental groups) and withholds the treatment from the other groups (control groups). The researcher thus intentionally alters the independent variable and subsequently observes the effect the direct intervention has had upon the control group or those subjects that did not receive the intentional intervention or treatment.

Control is the second criterion of experimental research and refers to the activities implemented by the researcher to eliminate all possible factors that could influence or affect the results of the independent or treatment variable on the dependent variable. Basically, control answers the question: Is there any other explanation that may be responsible for the resulting effects of the independent variable on the dependent variable? Although the control group or groups are the usual means of implementing control in experimental research, control may also be provided through the researcher's manipulation of variables, randomization, and the preparation of the experimental protocol or procedure.[15]

Randomization is the third criterion of experimental research and refers to the assignment of subjects to the experimental or control group(s) by the researcher on a random basis. Random selection of subjects infers that every subject in the proposed study has an equal chance of being assigned to any group. Equal chance, however, does not imply the same or like characteristics of the subjects. Randomization provides the most objective means by which equal representation of the sample may be attained. It is the only method of controlling the influence of possible extraneous variables.[16]

The strengths of experimental research are due to the power of control it affords over the relevant variables. Based on this control, experimental research provides the most objective and scientific means of testing cause and effect relationships and of providing the researcher the confidence by which causal relationships can be inferred. Causal statements, when supported by analysis of data, can conclude that the introduction of the independent variable, or X, made a difference based on the effects observed in the dependent variable, or Y. Experimental research enables the researcher to select those particular factors that will be most informative in relation to the research question being asked. The classical experimental design is shown in Figure 5–1.

The strengths of experimental research are also its weaknesses. Owing to the tightness of control required by the implementation of experimental research, it is extremely restrictive and artificial, particularly in real world situations where research frequently involves human subjects. Characteristics in human nature are difficult, if not impossible, to control. Patients/clients often behave in a different manner if their behavior is artificially restricted, manipulated, or exposed to systematic observation and

	Experimental Group	Control Group
Before Treatment		
After Treatment		

FIGURE 5–1
Classical experimental design.

evaluation.[17] Consideration of the ethical implications when the subjects are humans also inhibits the necessary manipulation required in experimental research. In addition, the highly controlled environment required for experimental research is not readily available in nursing. Based on the limitations inherent in the ability to conduct experimental research, true experimental research is seldom considered a viable means of research for clinical nursing research.

Although in the clinical setting true experimental research does not offer the nurse researcher the required environment to conduct research, a modification of the experimental type is available. This type of research is the field experiment. Field experiments incorporate the fundamental designs of the true experiment but are conducted in real world settings. Field experiments are, therefore, adaptable for use in the clinical areas. The field experiments, thus, will be developed with experimental and control groups and incorporate an independent variable that is manipulated by the researcher under controlled conditions in a lifelike setting.[18] The major advantage of field experiments are that the findings more closely approximate situations consistent with the real world. Field experiments, however, attempt to incorporate the strengths of the true experiment and are often self-limiting because of the researcher's inability to achieve control. Depending upon the research problem/question, field experiments, nevertheless, offer the nurse researcher a type of research that approximates to some degree the characteristics of the true experiment.

Quasi-Experimental Research

Quasi-experimental types of research and their accompanying designs can be implemented in social settings consistent with the real world. The purpose of these types of research is to approximate the conditions of experimental research in a setting that does not allow for the control and the manipulation of variables characteristic of experimental research.[19] The designs that accompany quasi-experimental research resemble closely the basic format found in experimental research designs but lack the features of control and randomization consistent with experimental designs.[20] Quasi-experimental types of research do, however, involve the manipulation of an independent variable or the introduction of a treatment characteristic of experimental research, but inferences of cause and effect relationships are extremely limited. To achieve the internal and external validity that is usually attainable with experimental research, compromises are necessary and require the introduction of compensatory controls by the researcher.

To compensate for the absence of either randomization and/or the control group's component, quasi-experimental research incorporates designs that provide for the collection of data over an extended period of time or designs that involve the use of pretesting. Although a variety of designs are available that incorporate extended time periods and pretesting formats, two such designs have become extremely useful to nurse researchers who conduct research in the clinical setting. These two quasi-experimental designs are referred to as the *nonequivalent control group pretest/posttest design* and the *time series design*. Since most of the following discussion is based on the work of Campbell and Stanley, and is limited in scope, the reader is encouraged to utilize this reference for additional coverage.[21]

Nonequivalent Control Group. Nonequivalent control group pretest/posttest designs resemble to a significant extent the pretest/posttest designs used in experimental research. The major difference between the two designs is the randomly assigned treatment groups used in experimental research. This difference is shown by the symbolic representation of the nonequivalent control group pretest/posttest design and the pretest/posttest experimental design found in Figures 5–2 and 5–3, respectively. The R (randomization) in Figure 5–3 denotes the difference.

To illustrate the use of a quasi-experimental control group pretest/posttest design a

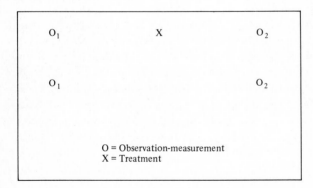

$$O_1 \qquad X \qquad O_2$$

$$O_1 \qquad\qquad O_2$$

O = Observation-measurement
X = Treatment

FIGURE 5–2
Nonequivalent control group pretest-posttest quasi-experimental design.

$$R \quad O_1 \qquad X \qquad O_2$$

$$R \quad O_1 \qquad\qquad O_2$$

R = Randomization
O = Observation-measurement
X = Treatment

FIGURE 5–3
Pretest-posttest experimental design.

discussion of this design is indicated. A nursing service department in a community hospital has decided to determine the nurses' satisfaction with the introduction of primary nursing care. The introduction of this plan of care will affect all nurses employed in the selected hospital, and thus the use of randomly assigned treatment groups required of the experimental design is not feasible. However, to determine the nurses' satisfaction with primary nursing care, another hospital with similar characteristics that has no plans of using primary nursing care could be chosen. Following the administration of a staff satisfaction questionnaire to both hospitals, baseline data could be obtained. After primary care nursing has been introduced in the first hospital and the nursing staff has had the opportunity of using this health delivery system for a predetermined amount of time, the staff satisfaction questionnaire would then be administered to the nurses of both hospitals. A difference reflected in the pretest/posttest questionnaire of both hospital groups would indicate the degree of satisfaction with the introduction of primary care nursing. This degree of satisfaction with the introduction of primary care nursing, however, would be valid only if no other inducements to staff satisfaction, such as salary increases, decreased working hours, or paid continuing educational expenses, were provided during the time of the study. This design does not offer the power offered by an experimental design, but some confidence in the results could be inferred if the nurses of both hospitals reflected similar answers on the pretest questionnaire.

Time Series Designs.   Time series designs allow for data collection over an extended period of time and the introduction of an experimental treatment during the course of the data collection period.[22] These designs are frequently used for a small number of subjects or single-subject research and are concerned not only with the resulting effects of the treatment introduced but also the behavioral process.[23] A symbolic representation of a time series design is shown in Figure 5–4. The reader will note that this design does not involve a control group or randomization. Although the features of a control group and randomization are lacking in the time series design, the extended observational times

FIGURE 5–4
Quasi-experimental time series design.

$$O_1 \quad O_2 \quad O_3 \quad O_4 \quad X \quad O_5 \quad O_6 \quad O_7 \quad O_8$$

O = Observations-Measurements
    (prior to treatment X, 1-4,
    after treatment X, 5-8)
X = Treatment

are incorporated into the design to increase the assurances that any change can be attributed to the introduction of the treatment. For example, if a research study was proposed to determine the impact of nurses working twelve-hour shifts on patient safety, a series of observations or measurements would be taken prior to the introduction of the twelve-hour shift. After the introduction of the twelve-hour shift another series of observations would be made. Based on the observations of patient safety prior to and after the introduction of the twelve-hour shift, the effects of the twelve-hour shift on patient safety could be determined. The number of observations required of the time series design (over an extended period of time) nullify significantly other variables that might be considered responsible for affecting the results. Time series designs offer the nurse researcher a tool by which research can be conducted without the necessity of having a control group and introducing randomization. In addition, these designs that use a small number of subjects or single-subject research provide the economy of both time and effort without negating the planning, implementing, and reporting essential to the research process.[24]

Nonequivalent control group pretest/posttest design and the time series design are two of many quasi-experimental research designs that lack the high degree of internal and external validity characteristic of experimental research. The researcher, therefore, when using quasi-experimental designs must be constantly aware that there may be other explanations for the results obtained. These other explanations are referred to as *threats to internal validity* or *plausible rival hypotheses* and include mortality, history, maturation, testing, selection, and instrumentation.[25] The definitions of each of these terms is as follows:

- *Mortality*. The differential loss of subjects from the group being compared to the group receiving the treatment.
- *History*. An event experienced by the subject besides the exposure of the treatment that affects the comparison.
- *Maturation*. The effect of the subject's responses caused by biological or psychological processes.
- *Testing*. The effects of a pretest upon the scores of a posttest.
- *Selection*. Pretreatment differences between the experimental and control groups.
- *Instrumentation*. Alterations occurring in the tools used for testing, including changes in human raters, or interviewers.

Strengths of quasi-experimental types of research are the practicality they offer, the feasibility of implementation, and an acceptable degree of generalizability. Quasi-experimental types of research and their accompanying designs, therefore, offer the nurse researcher an avenue for conducting research in the clinical setting not provided through the use of the experimental designs.

Weaknesses of quasi-experimental research are many, but to the extent the researcher can provide control the weaknesses can be limited. The weaknesses of these designs include the limited ability of the researcher to provide control, the minimal degree to which causal inferences can be made, and the compromises to internal validity.

Ex Post Facto Research

Ex post facto research studies are similar to experimental and quasi-experimental designs in structural characteristics and design development.[26] The discussion of ex post facto research is, therefore, indicated at this point in relation to the research continuum presented in Chapter 1. The term ex post facto means "from after the fact" and refers to that type of research that is conducted after variations in the independent variable have occurred. Examination of the independent variable is, thus, done retrospectively. The researcher begins with the dependent variable and retrospectively or after the fact studies the independent variables for their possible effects on the dependent variable.[27] The purpose of ex post facto research is to determine the relationship among variables. Since the independent variable has occurred as a natural event in the past, it cannot be manipulated as inherently characteristic of experimental research. Random assignment of subjects is, in addition, not possible. Thus, the major difference between experimental research and ex post facto research is control, which limits the researcher's ability to make inferences of causal relationships.[28] For an example, the researcher may wish to determine the self-esteem of thirty-five-year-old women who have been primarily in nursing service for the past ten years and those of thirty-five-year-old women who have occupied positions in nursing education during the same time period. The type of experience or the independent variable cannot be manipulated. The researcher would, thus, select subjects in whom the two aspects of the independent variable could be identified. The relationship between the variables, the type of experience, and self-esteem would, subsequently, be examined.

In ex post facto research it is impossible for the researcher to assign subjects at random or to assign treatments to groups at random. Based on this fact, a significant characteristic of ex post facto research is *self-selection*. Self-selection occurs when members of the groups being studied are in the groups, in part, because they differentially possess traits or characteristics extraneous to the research problem, characteristics that possibly influence or are otherwise related to the variables of the research problem.[29]

Correlational research is sometimes considered a form of ex post facto research. It, too, seeks to determine relationships among variables when the independent variable is not under the control of the researcher. Correlational research employs the use of an index that correlates the extent to which two variables are determined to be interrelated. Thus, hypertension may be positively correlated with high cholesterol diets, but the relationship of these two variables does not imply that high cholesterol diets cause hypertension. A functional relationship may be demonstrated among variables in correlational research studies, but causal or cause and effect relationships cannot be inferred.

A strength of ex post facto research is its ability to determine relationships among variables that have the potential of supporting causal relationships. Ex post facto research is also characteristic of the real world, and thus the results may have greater acceptance of generalizability than those research studies employing experimental designs. Weaknesses of post facto research are: (1) the inability to manipulate the independent variables, (2) the lack of power to randomize, and (3) the risk of improper interpretation.[30]

Descriptive Research

The use of descriptive types of research plays an important role in the advancement of nursing as a profession. Before a body of knowledge can be developed and experimental hypotheses tested, variables and their relationship to other variables must be described.[31] Descriptive types of research and their respective designs serve this purpose. In addition to describing variables, descriptive research compares groups of subjects in relation to an identified dependent variable, demonstrates correlations between two or more variables, and may predict behavior on the basis of what is known about one or more other variables.[32] Descriptive research is *present* oriented, as its primary function characterizes variables as they currently exist.

Descriptive research may or may not have an hypothesis. Subjects included in descriptive designs cannot be randomly selected to different groups, and, therefore, inferences of causal relationships, characteristic of experimental research, cannot be made. Descriptive research can describe phenomena but cannot provide any explanations.

The term *descriptive research* is sometimes categorized or classified by different authors in varying ways. In this text, descriptive research will refer to those researchable questions that are present oriented, provide data that are measurable, and have as their primary objective the accurate description of the characteristics of individuals, situations, or groups of individuals with emphasis upon frequency of occurrence. The three major descriptive research designs that will be discussed are survey, comparative, and correlational. The goal of each is to provide an accurate description of the variables in order to answer the proposed research question.

Survey Design. The survey design that is frequently referred to in the literature as descriptive survey research is one of the most widely used and oldest research designs. The survey usually involves a method of obtaining facts and figures in an attempt to describe a condition or learn the current status of something.[33] Frequently, the survey study is referred to as a sample survey, as it reflects a chosen sample of the population in which the discovery of the relative incidence, distribution, and interrelationships of sociological and psychological variables are the objective.[34] Questionnaires and interviews are the usual means of obtaining data for survey designs, although telephone surveys are becoming more widely used.

The most effective means of collecting data for descriptive/survey research is the interview. The interview technique involves the use of trained interviewers, who meet with their subjects and secure information from them in response to a predetermined set of questions. This set of questions is referred to as the *interview schedule,* and it consists of specific carefully developed questions that are designed to answer the research question. Interview technique is discussed in detail in Chapter 6.

Although surveys have as their primary objective the description of variables, many descriptive/survey designs prove to have far-reaching implications for action and change. Many changes in nursing education and nursing service have been made based on the results of survey designs that have been developed to determine existing attitudes, opinions, and facts. Surveys may be applied to many different populations and include a large range of topics. The topics may range from the brand of appliances used in the household to opinions reflecting preferences on national issues.

The survey design has limitations. These limitations include the superficiality of information that is received, the lack of confidence the researcher can infer from the relationship of variables that are examined, and the demand placed on personnel in relation to time and energy. The amount of information, however, that can be generated from either the use of small or large surveys that are well developed and constructed may justify the use of descriptive survey research designs.

An example of the simple survey design is found in Figure 5–5. This survey represents a questionnaire that was developed by a state nurses' association to determine the preference of its members as to selected options of implementing mandatory continuing education. The design illustrates a single box that represents the membership, a D indicating demographic data of the individual members, and a P representing the member's preference of the means for implementation. Data analysis in Figure 5–5 is done by frequency of responses converted to percentages (see Chapter 7). Figure 5–5 is one of the more simplistic of survey designs. Survey designs, however, may be significantly more complex.

Occasionally, researchers use a means of measurement similar to those used in sample surveys to determine variations in the subjects' responses over periods of time. These survey designs are called *longitudinal studies,* and they may have time intervals ranging from days to years. The purpose of longitudinal studies is to examine the subjects' responses over a period of time to detect possible emerging trends or developing issues. Longitudinal studies basically reflect a description of changes or differences. The data collected is analyzed by comparison statistical procedures.

Comparative Designs. Comparative designs compare levels or categories of an independent variable that usually cannot be manipulated experimentally on some dependent variable for which it is hypothesized that differences exist.[35] The responses to some questions asked of subjects may be compared to certain characteristics of the subjects. These characteristics may include age, sex, educational level, socioeconomic status, diagnosis, or level of understanding. For example, the continuing education department in a large metropolitan university hospital sponsored a clinical decision-making in-service education program. The participants were compared on the basis of

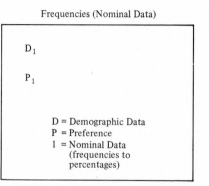

Frequencies (Nominal Data)

D_1

P_1

D = Demographic Data
P = Preference
1 = Nominal Data
  (frequencies to
  percentages)

FIGURE 5–5
Sample survey design.

whether they had experienced a formalized research course (independent variable). The dependent variables include: B—beliefs about decision-making nursing practice, U— use of decision making in practice, and K—knowledge of decision-making principles. The participants were asked to complete a questionnaire that assessed beliefs, usage, and knowledge of decision making as well as demographic data and whether the subjects had had a formalized research course. The groups of questionnaires were then compared with the other variables. The results of the comparisons indicate the differences between those participants who had had a research course and those who had not. The design developed for this descriptive comparative research is referred to as an *intact group comparison design*. It is shown in Figure 5–6. The reader will note that although differences may be demonstrated by the group of participants who had had a formalized course in research, it cannot be inferred that the research course was responsible for change reflected in the dependent variables.

Correlational Designs.   Correlational research designs have been briefly discussed in relation to the similarities they share with ex post facto research designs. In addition to the ability of correlational studies to indicate relationships among variables and the extent to which these variables are related, the magnitude and the direction of variables may also be determined. The magnitude and the direction of the relationship is determined by a correlational index and at times may demonstrate a significant positive or negative relationship. Correlations that are deemed significant frequently become the basis from which hypotheses are generated and subsequently tested through experimental research. Several correlational designs are available to the researcher; however, only the simple correlational design will be presented. An example of the simple correlational design might be a hypothesized relationship between patient compliance with a diabetic regimen and scheduled follow-up visits in the home by communi-

FIGURE 5–6
Intact group comparison design.

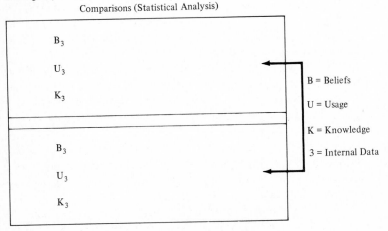

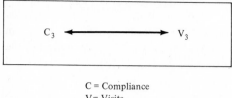

Correlational (Statistical Analysis)

C = Compliance
V = Visits
3 = Interval Data

FIGURE 5–7
Simple correlational design.

ty health nurses. This relationship is shown in Figure 5–7. The design illustrates an enclosed two-directional arrow in which C represents compliance and V nurse visits. Data retrieved would be assessed according to interval data analysis (see Chapter 7).

The scope of descriptive types of research varies from simplistic designs to those that are highly sophisticated and complex. Each design is intended to answer the question: What is/are the relationships between or among the variables? The purpose of all descriptive designs is an accurate description of the variables.

Historical Research

The historical type of research, or historiography, is the art and science of reconstructing the past from a critical view of documents, artifacts, literature, and accounts of eyewitnesses or participants of the event.[36] Historical research seeks to search the past but also to relate events that occurred in the past to current and future developments. The researcher involved in historical research critically examines events of the past, weighs the evidence in relation to the validity of past sources, and interprets the evidence.[37] The process involved in conducting historical research is thus similar to that of other types of research. Significant differences, however, exist.

Historical research begins with a particular identified problem of interest. Hypotheses, however, are not usually identified as explicitly as in other types of research, but instead resemble broadly stated hunches that relate to relationships between natural events, trends, and phenomena.

The major requirement that is expected of the historical researcher is the use of *primary* sources from which data is gathered. *Primary sources* of data include such items as an original record of a significant occasion, minutes of an important organization, or an eyewitness account of a particular event. *Secondary sources* of data, in contrast, refer to reports of events, such as newspapers or narrative summaries that have been modified by transmission from one person to another. For example, if a researcher wanted to examine the significant events surrounding Florence Nightingale and her attempts to lay the foundation for nursing in London, access to diaries and written accounts of the participants involved in those events would be indicated.

The advantage of conducting historical research includes the opportunity of the researcher to examine incidents or events with the advantage of elapsed time and the subsequent development of a more objective perspective. In addition, the historical researcher can use previous research as a reference, and because records and data are available there is no need to develop data-gathering instruments. Despite these advantages, the historical data collected by the researcher must survive tests of validity and reliability in a well-prescribed manner to establish truth and avoid distortion.[38] The criteria that ensure the validity and reliability of historical research are external criticism and internal criticism. External criticism refers to the *validity* of data sources, while internal criticism asks whether the content of the data sources reflects the *true meaning*.

Disadvantages inherent in conducting historical research involve the difficulty often experienced by the researcher in locating primary sources of data. Control over existing documents, records, and artifacts is extremely limited. In addition, only those records that have survived time may be used in data collection, and thus the possibility of bias exists. Despite these disadvantages the value of historical research is becoming well recognized by nurses, as it offers an avenue by which professional identity may be enhanced. An understanding of the historical aspects of nursing is conducive to establishing a comprehensive definition of nursing and provides a means by which new and expanded roles for nurses may develop. The value of historical research is currently being well documented, as evidenced by an increase in this type of research in the literature.

Field Research Studies (Nonexperimental Research)

Field studies, or field research, is an inductive scientific mode of inquiry directed toward discovering relations and interactions among sociological, psychological, or educational variables in real social situations.[39] Problems of social structure or specific phenomena that relate to ongoing social situations are subsequently well suited to field methodology.[40] Field research permits one to seek what is, rather than predict relations, and considering all research methods open to researchers, field studies are the closest to real life.[41] The use of field research methods is particularly appropriate to nurse researchers, as they are conducive to implementation in the practice area and allow investigative activities of subjects in the real world. A variety of practice areas may be used to conduct field studies and include the hospital, the outpatient clinic, nursing homes, and community health agencies. Subjects can be patients, families, and health team members.

According to Katz, field research studies may be divided into two groups—exploratory field studies and hypothesis-testing studies.[42] Exploratory studies have three major purposes: to discover significant variables in the field situation, to discover relations among variables, and to lay the groundwork for later, more systematic and rigorous testing of hypotheses.[43] Qualitative data is usually generated through the use of exploratory field studies. Hypothesis-testing research involves preliminary activities related to method and measurement that need solidification by the researcher prior to implementing studies designed to test a hypothesis.

Field studies involve a humanistic and pragmatic approach within a dynamic and changing environment. The inherent complexities of field studies are, therefore, inconsistent with the controlled or partially controlled format of many other types of research. Manipulation of an independent variable by the researcher rarely occurs.

Exploratory field studies require the researcher to develop a general problem area for investigation. This problem area is referred to as the problem focus. Once the data collection is begun, the researcher devises a system by which the data are organized. The results are, subsequently, weighed and analyzed. Conclusions are derived in an objective manner. Results of the exploration frequently provide new leads to the initial focus, solidify the research question, or generate new hypotheses.

The primary methods used to collect data in field research are the *interview* and *observation*. Although the *interview* will be discussed more fully in Chapter 6, its vital role in field research warrants some additional comments here. Because the majority of data generated by field studies is qualitative in nature, the unstructured interview is commonly used. The unstructured interview provides the respondents an opportunity to elaborate upon the questions posed by the researcher. Questions that are inductively constructed such as what, why, and how are indicated. These questions, however, must be consistent with the problem focus in order that the researcher may more narrowly define the problem under investigation. The researcher, therefore, who uses the interview format must be skilled in the process of interviewing.

The second method used to collect data in field studies is through the use of *observation*. Observation in field studies is accomplished by two field study techniques, observation and participant observation. The technique of observation requires that the researcher observe the setting or situation consistent with the problem focus. Participant observation refers to both the observer and participant roles employed by the researcher in the setting or situation dictated by the problem under study (see Chapter 6).

The strengths of field studies are realism, the significance of the findings, and the strength of the variables. The weaknesses of field studies are its ex post facto characteristics, and the lack of precise measurement tools. Practical problems such as cost, time, and feasibility are also potential concerns.

In addition to exploratory and hypothesis-testing field studies, field research that employs the sociological concept of grounded theory is currently being viewed as significant to professional nursing. Field research that employs grounded theory is inductive in nature and is directed toward the generation of qualitative data. Grounded theory refers to the production of theory by a direct ongoing comparative analysis of data.[44] Comparative analysis involves the concurrent collection, collation, and analysis of data. Theory derived by this process is considered "grounded" by the data. Analysis of data is accomplished through the constant comparative method that employs a systematic method of organizing "core categories" and their particular properties. Core categories are the central themes that evolve from similarly perceived properties of the retrieved data that are identified and named by the researcher (see Table 8–2).

To date, the use of grounded theory has resulted in a number of significant studies that are directly related to nursing practice. Studies that have explored awareness of dying, pain management, and stepfather families have used the concept of grounded theory in the generation of new knowledge required in situations nurses are confronted with daily.

Strengths of grounded theory are the characteristics that suggest its use as theory for practice. These strengths are the ease of understanding, the fit with the real world, general practicality, and the partial control it offers the user over daily situations characterized by change. Lack of objectivity by the researcher is viewed as a weakness of grounded theory.

Case Studies

A case study is a thorough in-depth analysis of an individual, group, institution, or other social unit. The case study method may be used to test hypotheses, but more frequently the aim is exploration. Problems for case study investigation may be broadly or narrowly defined. Methods of data collection include records, artifacts, or observation, but the method most commonly used is the interview, which provides a means of generating qualitative data. The results of case studies are in-depth insights to individual problems in a naturalistic setting.

Case studies in nursing are usually concerned with the development of a comprehensive picture of the variables, directly related to the patient/clients' history, care, or condition. Collection of data frequently includes the patient/clients' present status, past history, situational, and environmental factors.

Nurses in the clinical setting are often confronted with unique patient situations that warrant in-depth assessments or analysis. Nursing interventions are also amenable to comprehensive analysis and evaluation. Situations such as these are good sources for case studies. An example of a case study might be the patient who has had a myocardial infarction and is not progressing despite a "normal" physiological postinfarct status. This situation offers the nurse an opportunity to undertake an in-depth analysis consistent with the case study method. The strength of case studies is the in-depth analysis that they produce. Findings from case studies frequently increase nurses' understanding and expand their base of knowledge. Weaknesses of case studies are their lack of generalizability and subjectivity.

SUMMARY

Types of research and their respective designs are derived from the three major categories of research that resemble the broad methodological approaches. The methodological approaches are, thus, experimental, quasi-experimental, and field research studies (nonexperimental). Each approach is characterized by the type of thinking employed in problem formulation, the setting, where the research is to be conducted, and the type of data expected to be generated.

The pilot study is a miniversion of the major research study and provides a trial run of the study in preparation for conducting the proposed study. Its purpose is to detect any potential difficulties that need to be corrected prior to the implementation of the research study.

Experimental research is the most scientific of all research, as it provides for control through manipulation, randomization, and control group assignment. Experimental research, however, requires a highly controlled environment and lacks the realism and practicability of methods that are particularly appropriate for use in the real world. The field experiment approximates the classical experimental design and is used to some success in the real world; however, it is limited, as control is difficult to achieve.

Quasi-experimental types of research and their accompanying designs are conducive to implementation in the real world. The introduction of controls such as pretesting and extended time periods by the researcher is required, however, to ensure internal and external validity. Two quasi-experimental types of research, the nonequivalent control group pretest/posttest design and the time series design, were discussed as being particularly useful to nurse researchers. Threats to internal validity or plausible rival hypotheses may occur with the use of quasi-experimental research methods. The researcher, therefore, needs to be consistently aware of this possibility. Strengths of quasi-experimental research are the practicality they offer, the feasibility of implementation, and an acceptable degree of generalizability. Weaknesses of quasi-experimental research are the lack of control they offer, the minimal degree to which causal inferences can be made, and the compromises to internal validity.

Ex post facto research is similar to experimental and quasi-experimental designs in structural characteristics and design development. Ex post facto research refers to the type of research that is conducted after variations in the independent variable have occurred. The purpose of ex post facto research is to determine the relationship among the variables. A strength of ex post facto research is the ability to determine relationships between variables that potentially support causal relationships. Lack of control is the major weakness of ex post facto research. Self-selection is an inherent characteristic of ex post facto research designs.

Descriptive types of research include survey, longitudinal, comparison, and correlational research studies. The major purpose of descriptive research is to accurately describe the variables. The survey is the most widely used and oldest of the descriptive types of research. The survey usually involves a method of obtaining facts and figures in an attempt to describe a condition or learn the current status of something. The survey frequently employs the use of the questionnaire. Surveys may be applied to many populations and includes a large range of topics. Comparative designs compare levels or categories of an independent variable that cannot usually be manipulated on some dependent variable for which a hypothesis indicates that differences exist. Correlational research designs resemble ex post facto research, as they indicate relationships among the variables. The magnitude and the direction of the relationship may also be determined through the use of a correlational index.

Historical research reconstructs the past from a critical view of documents, artifacts, literature, and eyewitness accounts. This type of research seeks to search the past but also to relate events that have occurred to current and future developments. The use of primary sources of data is a major requirement of conducting historical research.

Field research is an inductive scientific mode of inquiry directed toward discovering relations and interactions among sociological, psychological, or educational variables in social situations. The use of field research is advantageous to nurse researchers, as it permits one to seek "what is" and is the closest of all research methods to reality. Field research studies consist of two types, exploratory and hypothesis testing. Both types are directed toward exploration or solidification of a potential researchable problem. Qualitative data is usually sought through the use of field studies. The concept of grounded theory is a recent development in field research methods. This sociological method of scientific inquiry employs inductive thinking and generates qualitative data. Grounded theory refers to the production of theory by a direct ongoing comparative analysis of data. Data are collected through the process of unstructured interview techniques. Use of grounded theory has expanded the knowledge base of professional nursing practice. The major strength of grounded theory is its practice base orientation.

The case study research method is a thorough in-depth analysis of an individual, group, institution, or other social unit. Case studies in nursing are conducted to provide a comprehensive picture of variables that relate to the patients/clients' history, care, or condition. The results of case studies frequently increase the professional's understanding and expand her or his knowledge base.

QUESTIONS FOR STUDY AND DISCUSSION

1 Explain the types of research and their respective designs in relation to the research continuum.

2 Name three advantages of conducting a pilot study.

3 Define the purpose of experimental research design.

4 Discuss the inherent weaknesses of experimental research.

5 Compare and contrast experimental and quasi-experimental types of research.

6 Explain the compromises of control and randomization offered by the quasi-experimental time series design.

7 Describe survey, comparative, and correlational descriptive research.

8 Name four possible threats to internal validity commensurate with the use of quasi-experimental designs.

9 Discuss the similarities and differences of experimental and ex post facto research designs.

10 Design a research study that incorporates the use of the survey/descriptive design.

11 Explain the potential problems in the use of historical research.

12 Name the conditions under which field research studies might be considered an appropriate methodology.

13 Differentiate the type of data generated through experimental, quasi-experimental research, and field research studies.

14 Explain the potential value of the concept of grounded theory to professional nursing practice.

REFERENCES

1 Donna Schantz, and Carol A. Lindeman, "The Research Design," *Journal of Nursing Administration*, vol. 12, no. 1, 1982, p. 35.

2 Clifford J. Drew, *Introduction to Designing Research and Evaluation*, Mosby, St. Louis, 1976, p. 34.

3 Schantz and Lindeman, loc. cit.

4 Sonya I. Shelly, *Research Methods in Nursing and Health*, Little, Brown, Boston, 1984, p. 14.

5 Denise F. Polit, and Bernadette P. Hungler, *Nursing Research: Principles and Methods*, 2d ed., Lippincott, Philadelphia, 1983, p. 609.

6 Stephen Isaac, and William B. Michael, *Handbook in Research and Evaluation*, Edits Publishers, San Diego, 1983, p. 34.

7 Sydney D. Krampitz, and Natalie Pavlovich, *Readings for Nursing Research*, Mosby, St. Louis, 1981, p. 49.

8 Norma G. McHugh, and Jean E. Johnson, "Clinical Nursing Research: Beyond the Methods Books," *Nursing Outlook,* vol. 8, no. 6, 1980, p. 355.

9 Krampitz and Pavlovich, op. cit., pp. 50–51.

10 Eleanor Walters Treece, and James William Treece, Jr., *Elements of Research in Nursing,* 3d ed., Mosby, St. Louis, 1982, p. 176.

11 Fred N. Kerlinger, *Foundations of Behavioral Research,* 2d ed., Holt, Rinehart, and Winston, 1973, p. 315.

12 Krampitz and Pavlovich, op. cit., p. 67.

13 Isaac and Michael, op. cit., p. 52.

14 Polit and Hungler, op. cit., p. 142.

15 Polit and Hungler, op. cit., p. 143.

16 Pamela J. Brink, and Marilyn J. Wood, *Basic Steps in Planning Nursing Research from Question to Proposal,* 2d ed., Wadsworth Health Sciences Division, Monterey, California, 1983, p. 98.

17 Isaac and Michael, op. cit., p. 153.

18 Mary Ann Sweeney, and Peter Olivieri, *An Introduction to Nursing Research,* Lippincott, Philadelphia, 1981, p. 117.

19 Isaac and Michael, op. cit., p. 54.

20 Polit and Hungler, op. cit., p. 154.

21 Donald T. Campbell, and Julian C. Stanley, *Experimental and Quasi-Experimental Designs for Research,* Rand McNally, Chicago, 1963, pp. 34–56.

22 Polit and Hungler, op. cit., p. 158.

23 Drew, op. cit., p. 38.

24 Karyn Holin, "Single Subject Research," *Nursing Research,* vol. 32, no. 4, 1983, pp. 253–255.

25 Campbell and Stanley, op. cit., pp. 13–16.

26 Polit and Hungler, op. cit., p. 170.

27 Krampitz and Pavlovich, op. cit., p. 67.

28 Kerlinger, op. cit., p. 380.

29 Kerlinger, op. cit., p. 381.

30 Kerlinger, op. cit., p. 390.

31 Shelley, op. cit., p. 89.

32 Shelley, op. cit., p. 89.

33 Catherine H. C. Seaman, and Phyllis J. Verhonick, *Research Methods,* 2d ed., Appleton-Century-Crofts, Norwalk, Connecticut, 1982, p. 34.

34 Kerlinger, op. cit., p. 110.

35 Shelley, op. cit., p. 90.

36 Krampitz and Pavlovich, op. cit., p. 54.

37 Kerlinger, op. cit., p. 701.

38 Theresa A. Christy, "The Methodology of Historical Research: A Brief Introduction," *Nursing Research,* vol. 24, no. 3, 1975, pp. 190–191.

39 Kerlinger, op. cit., p. 405.

40 Leonard Schatzman, and Anselm L. Strauss, *Field Research,* Prentice-Hall, Englewood Cliffs, New Jersey, 1973, p. 21.

41 Kerlinger, op. cit., p. 407.

42 David Katz, "Field Studies," in Leon Festinger and David Katz (eds.), *Research Methods in the Behavioral Sciences,* Holt, Rinehart, and Winston, New York, 1953, pp. 75–83.

43 Kerlinger, op. cit., pp. 407–408.

44 Barney G. Glaser, and Anselm L. Strauss, *The Discovery of Grounded Theory: Strategies for Qualitative Research*, Aldine, Chicago, 1967, p. 32.

BIBLIOGRAPHY

Abdellah, Faye G., and Eugene Levine, *Better Patient Care Through Nursing Research*, Macmillan, New York, 1965.

Blalock, Hubert M., *An Introduction to Social Research*, Prentice-Hall, Englewood Cliffs, New Jersey, 1970.

Dempsey, Patricia Ann, and Arthur D. Dempsey. *The Research Process in Nursing*, Van Nostrand, New York, 1981.

Diers, Donna, *Research in Nursing Practice*, Lippincott, Philadelphia, 1979.

Downs, Florence, *A Source Book of Nursing Research*, 3d ed., Davis, Philadelphia, 1984.

Downs, Florence S., and Margaret A. Newman, *A Source Book of Nursing Research*, 2d ed., Davis, Philadelphia, 1977.

Fagerhaugh, Claire, and Anselm L. Strauss, *Politics of Pain Management*, Addison-Wesley, Menlo Park, California, 1977.

Fox, David J., *Fundamentals of Research in Nursing*, 4th ed., Appleton-Century-Crofts, New York, 1982.

Glaser, Barney G., *Theoretical Sensitivity Advances in the Methodology of Grounded Theory*, Sociology Press, Mill Valley, California, 1978.

Glaser, Barney G., and Anselm L. Strauss, *Awareness of Dying*. Aldine, Chicago, 1965.

Glaser, Barney G., and Anselm L. Strauss: "The Purpose and Credibility of Qualitative Research," *Nursing Research*, vol. 15, no. 1, 1966, pp. 56–61.

Krueger, Janelle C., Allen H. Nelson, and Mary Opal Wolanin, *Nursing Research Development, Collaboration, and Utilization*, Aspen Systems, Germantown, Maryland, 1978.

Seltz, Claire, Maria Johoda, Morton Deutsch, and Stuart W. Cook: *Research Methods in Social Relations*, Holt, Rinehart, and Winston, New York, 1959.

Simon, Julian L., *Basic Research Methods in Social Science*, Random House, New York, 1969.

Stern, Phyllis N., "Grounded Theory Methodology: Its Uses and Processes," *Image: The Journal of Nursing Scholarship*, vol. 12, no. 1, 1980, pp. 20–23.

CHAPTER 6

COLLECTION OF DATA

After the research problem/question has been clearly defined, the literature searched, and the methodology determined, one of the most interesting and challenging phases for many researchers begins. This part of the study often involves direct contact with the subjects/patients/clients in a clinical setting. For the nurse who finds direct patient contact one of the most satisfying parts of nursing, this phase is often welcomed after a long period of reading, studying, planning, and writing the research proposal.

The researcher soon discovers, however, that there is much more involved in the collection of data than simply deciding how and where to collect the data. The process involves determining the most appropriate method to collect the data, selecting the subjects, and requesting the various approvals the researcher must obtain before the process of data collection may begin.

GENERAL CONSIDERATIONS OF DATA COLLECTION

Before deciding upon a specific method of data collection, there are several general factors related to this process that should be considered. Most important, data need to be collected that will answer the research question(s). Additional data that are of interest may be collected at the same time and may help to explain the other data collected, but the researcher needs to remember that the primary purpose of the data collection is to answer the research question(s). Quite often additional data will raise new research questions that may be as important or more important than the original research question.

As the method of data collection is being selected, it needs to be determined exactly how and to what extent the data will be summarized and analyzed. A relatively short questionnaire, for example, may be simple to construct based on the research question(s). However, the researcher must plan how the data will be used. For example,

- Can the responses be categorized and/or summarized in some way so that analysis of the data is possible?
  - Will the analysis provide adequate data to make conclusions from the results?
  - Will the conclusions answer the research question(s)?

There are many questions that the researcher must recognize while determining the method of data collection.

MAJOR METHODS OF DATA COLLECTION

The method of data collection chosen must be appropriate for the research problem/question and the research design. Beginning researchers will also want to evaluate carefully which methods they will use, considering time required, funds that may be needed, their own capabilities, available consultation and/or other assistance to help with the process, and the type, availability, and number of subjects to be chosen for the study. These factors will be discussed as the various methods are presented.

The methods to be presented in this chapter include:

- Observation
- Questionnaires
- Interviews
- Physical data
- Records and reports
- Standardized scales and tests

Observation

The nurse has learned the importance of observation in implementing the nursing process. The skill of observation is an essential part of nursing practice. The importance of observation was discussed in Chapter 3 as one cue to researchable problems. Accurate, objective, and systematic observation, however, as required in the collection of data for research, is not an easy task.

Structured Observation. If the design of the study utilizes the deductive approach, the researcher will usually use a structured format. Structured observation involves a list of specific predetermined behaviors that will be observed and recorded on a prepared observation record. The preparation of an observation guide or an observation checklist may be a good place to begin. A structured technique of this type will help the researcher to identify clearly exactly what is to be observed based on the research question.

Perhaps the researcher wants to evaluate a child's reaction to the way a nurse approaches the child to give an intramuscular injection. Or the nurse might want to observe the amount of time specific categories of nursing staff spend in the rooms of terminally ill patients. In the first situation, the researcher will need to decide exactly which type of behaviors of the child should be observed and which type of behaviors of the nurse should be observed. In the second situation, the researcher may simply want to observe over a period of several days how many times registered nurses, licensed vocational (practical) nurses, and nurse aides enter terminally ill patients' rooms and how long each one stays in the room during selected hours. A sample of a structured observation guide for the last situation will be found in Table 6–1. As can be noted, even a relatively simple situation requires a careful plan.

Unstructured Observation.   Using the unstructured observation, the researcher must be acutely aware of the parameters of the situation to be observed, but he or she does not have a predetermined idea of what to expect. The researcher notes and records the behaviors of the patient for later summary during which these behaviors are grouped into several major classifications for analysis and interpretation. Unstructured observation may be utilized in a pilot study (observation of a few sample subjects) first and then the behaviors observed can be used to prepare a structured interview guide.[1]

Recording Observations.   Whether the structured or unstructured method is used, the researcher will need to plan some method of recording observations. These observations usually are recorded at the time of the behavior because the researcher cannot be expected to remember exactly what was observed. However, additional details should be recorded as soon as possible, which will help with later analysis. A tape recorder is often used for this process. The use of videotapes for the observation of patient behavior is ideal, if the proper consents are obtained and there are funds available to purchase the tapes.

Advantages of Observation.   This methodology is particularly relevant for descriptive studies, especially of patient behavior. Observation allows the researcher to study the real world; that is, nursing care and/or patient reaction and behavior at the time it is occurring. The practicing nurse may find this method particularly useful in small studies of nursing care problems on the unit. Except for the researcher's time spent in observation, the method is relatively inexpensive.

Disadvantages of Observation.   Observation is time consuming for the researcher, especially if collecting the data alone. The observer can only observe one patient and/or one situation at one time, thus possibly limiting the number of subjects who can be included in the study. If more than one observer is used, it is essential that they all observe exactly the same behaviors. Even when they have expert training in observing, individual experiential and/or cultural factors may affect their observations. Researcher subjectivity of any kind can hinder the objectivity of the observations. Skillful and objective observation is difficult, especially in a research situation that involves human behavior of two or more people. Because the subjects in the study, patients or personnel, must give their consent to be observed, the fact that they know that they are being observed for research purposes may influence their behavior and distort the results of the study. This problem is known as the *Hawthorne effect,* and although it also occurs with other methods of data collection, it is particularly a problem when direct observation is used. If the observer/researcher can help the subjects to be more comfortable and relaxed in the situation, however, the subjects will usually begin to act in a normal manner.[2]

TABLE 6.1
SAMPLE OF A SIMPLE STRUCTURED OBSERVATION GUIDE TO STUDY DIRECT CONTACT OF NURSES WITH TERMINALLY ILL HOSPITALIZED PATIENTS

Hospital Unit: 4 West
Date: 6/20/85

Time: 7 AM—11 AM
Observer: J. Jones

	Registered Nurses			Licensed Vocational Nurses			Nurse Aides		
Nurse	Nurse	#Xs Entered Room	Length of Stay (min)	Nurse	#Xs Entered Room	Length of Stay (min)	Nurse	#Xs Entered Room	Length of Stay (min)
Patient #1 #1	#1	1	5	#1	1	10	#1	1	30
#2	#2	1	2	#2	1	5	#2	1	5
Patient #2 #1	#1	1	2	#1	1	2	#1	1	15
				#2			#2	1	5

Another problem is the fact that the nurse/observer/researcher is sometimes tempted to become involved in nursing care because of the educational background and nature of the nurse. The participant/observer role is often used in field studies that seek qualitative data based on the inductive approach. The nurse may be observing and collecting data during the time that nursing care is being given. The inductive approach is discussed in more detail in Chapter 5.

Questionnaires

One of the most common methods used by beginning researchers is the questionnaire, probably because it is relatively easy to use and inexpensive. The items on the questionnaire should, of course, provide data that will answer the research question. Additional data *may* be requested (for example, demographic data such as age, sex, marital status, and religion) even though these data do not specifically relate to the research question. These types of data may be helpful in explaining the results later. It is better to include such data from the beginning of the study than to wish later that the data had been collected. However, the questionnaire should not be too long, so requests for irrelevant data should not be included.

Advantages of the Questionnaire.   Questionnaires are relatively easy to develop and distribute. This process usually allows for a larger sample from a wider geographical area and saves the researcher's time. Questionnaires may be handed out to groups of people at one time (for example, students in a class or patients in a clinic); mailed to individuals; distributed by other persons than the researcher (for example, the office nurse of selected physicians who consent to participate); or left in envelopes at patients' bedsides.

Because the questionnaire provides for more anonymity than observation or the interview, subjects may feel more free to respond with exactly what they think and feel, making the data more valid. Subjects usually complete the questionnaire in their own environment (home or hospital room) and are given a period of time to complete it and return it.

Disadvantages of the Questionnaire.   One of the advantages of the questionnaire is also a disadvantage. Because most questionnaires provide for anonymity, there is also the problem of the subject not understanding or misinterpreting the questions because the questionnaire is answered in complete privacy without the use of a name. Therefore, subjects may respond to the same question in completely different kinds of ways, thus making summary and analysis difficult and validity of the results questionable.

Another disadvantage of anonymity is the fact that the subject may not fill out or return the questionnaire, especially if it is mailed, thus making follow-up impossible. Many mailed questionnaires are discarded by the potential subjects. "A response rate greater than 50 percent is probably sufficient for most purposes,"[3] and an 80 to 90 percent return is considered exceptional. Each questionnaire can be coded in some way with the subject assured of confidentiality rather than anonymity so that follow-up is possible, but this process sometimes prevents the subject from giving true responses.

Still another disadvantage is the fact that the subjects who return the questionnaires may represent a biased sample. Would the 50 percent of the subjects who did not return the questionnaire have responded differently than the 50 percent who did? In order to encourage the highest return possible, the questionnaire should be as short, clear, and attractive as possible. Instructions for filling out the questionnaire should be very specific. A few examples are always helpful. An attractive color of paper and format often has a positive effect on potential subjects. Using both sides of one sheet of paper will make the questionnaire appear shorter. In most instances the questionnaire should be short enough so that subjects can complete it in thirty minutes or less.

Enclosing a stamped and self-addressed envelope with mailed questionnaires will usually increase the percent of return. A later follow-up postcard to all subjects thanking them for returning the questionnaire and asking them to do so if they have not will also usually increase the return rate. See Table 6-2 for a list of general factors to consider in developing a research questionnaire.

Interviews

The interview is somewhat similar to observation in that it involves direct contact with the subject, either in person or by telephone. The nurse has learned good communication skills and had experience doing health histories, so this method should be familiar. Effective communication skills are essential when using the interview method.

Just like a health history or a nursing history, there are many different types of interview formats. The interview may be structured, semistructured, or unstructured. The structured format involves the use of an interview guide with specific questions to ask the subject. The interview guide is developed so that the research question can be answered.

TABLE 6.2
GENERAL FACTORS TO CONSIDER IN DEVELOPING A RESEARCH QUESTIONNAIRE

- Limit the number of questions to the essential ones needed to answer the research question(s).
- Decide upon the type (format) of questions to be used; for example, structured, semistructured, open-ended.
- Write instructions for answering the questionnaire clearly and concisely.
- Prepare the questionnaire to appear as attractive (colored paper) and as short (use front and back of paper) as possible.
- Avoid the use of abbreviations, professional jargon, colloquial terms, slang, and words that denote sexism, racism, and ageism.
- Avoid leading, embarrassing, and biased questions.
- Plan the specific means of summarizing the answers and analyzing the results.
- Try out the preliminary form of the questionnaire with peers or colleagues to determine if the instructions and questions are clearly understood.

Telephone interviews are widely used by the business community for marketing research and by political groups for determining candidate preference, but they have not been used much in nursing. Telephone interviews could be used to evaluate a hospital discharge planning program, for example, or to assess the image of nursing in general or of a particular hospital in the community.

Advantages of the Interview Method.   Because there is face-to-face contact between the researcher and the subject, the researcher has the opportunity to clarify questions in order to obtain the most accurate data from the subject. As a part of this process, the researcher is alert to nonverbal as well as verbal communication. Also, because the researcher usually goes to the subject rather than vice versa, the subjects may feel more secure and comfortable in their own surroundings, even if it is a hospital room. Although the questionnaire may seem simpler to use because the subject can fill it out alone, more complete information is usually obtained with an interview because of the presence of the interviewer. A combination of questionnaire and interview is usually an effective method. The interview method can be used with both the deductive and inductive approach.

Disadvantages of the Interview Method.   The interview, like observation, is time consuming. Even if the researcher utilizes a structured approach, one cannot take a chance on hindering rapport with subjects and thus possibly losing important data by hurrying them or cutting them off. Sometimes interviews that are intended to be twenty to thirty minutes last for two or three hours. Although relevant data may be obtained, the time element limits the number of subjects who can be interviewed.

Physical Data

Some studies will require the collection of specific physical data from the patient. Physical assessment skills and experience will be very helpful if specific physical data need to be collected. These type of data may range from the very simple to the complex, such as those noted in the following list:

- Vital signs
- Skin color, warmth, character, texture, moisture, turgor, folds
- Pupillary size and constriction
- Hearing capabilities
- Laboratory tests, such as blood counts
- Electrocardiogram readings

For example, the simple procedure for taking a temperature has been studied by a number of nurse researchers. As noted in Chapter 2, many procedures in nursing have been based on tradition and intuition rather than scientific investigation. Several questions about procedures for taking oral temperatures have been raised by nurse researchers. Some of these are:

- How long does the thermometer need to be left in the mouth to obtain an accurate reading?

• When a patient has been smoking, drinking hot or cold liquids, or chewing gum before an oral temperature is taken, does it affect the temperature reading? If so, how long should the nurse wait before taking the oral temperature? One minute? Two minutes? Five minutes?

• At what age can a child have an oral rather than a rectal temperature taken?

• Should a nurse take the temperature orally or rectally in a patient who has had a heart attack in the last twenty-four hours or one who is receiving oxygen?

Some of these questions are being studied through the systematic collection and analysis of physical data.[4,5]

Records and Reports

In a descriptive or exploratory study, the nurse may want to review, summarize, and analyze specific written data. Examples of types of written material the nurse might need to review to answer specific research questions are:

• Patient records and charts (such as nurses' notes, surgery reports, or medication records)

• Incident or accident reports (for example, why do more incidents involving patients occur on one unit or one shift more than others?)

• Health screening data (for example, what is the relationship between dietary history and red blood cell count?)

• Vital statistics of a particular community, state, county, city, or census tract (for example, what is the relationship between family income and birth rate?)

• United States government census data (for example, why is the infant mortality rate higher in one census tract than another?)

If access to these records is readily available, this method of data collection is usually quite simple and inexpensive. Another advantage is the fact that human behavior is not a variable because there is no need for patient contact. Therefore, the researcher can record the data needed over time and in a quiet environment. The research is limited, however, to the data that are available.

Standardized Scales and Tests

If an instrument of some type is needed to measure one or more specific variables, *the beginning researcher should seek and use a standardized scale or test if at all possible.* A standardized instrument means that it has been tested and used with a large number of people in a variety of settings to determine its validity and reliability.

Validity.   Validity means the degree to which an instrument measures what it is supposed to measure. If the instrument does not measure what is intended, the results obtained from the data collected by the instrument will not answer the research question. The major types of validity are:

- Face
- Content
- Criterion
  Concurrent
  Predictive
- Construct

Face validity.   Face validity is the most basic kind of validity and is determined by researchers as they attempt to show that the concept being measured is clearly the same as the concept defined by the researcher. From personal knowledge of and experience with the concept, the measuring tool *appears* to measure the concept. "Face validity, if properly used, . . . can be a powerful tool. The power of face validity is determined largely by the power of the logic and arguments used by the researcher to claim face validity."[6] If beginning researchers plan to develop their own measuring instrument, they should, at the least, attempt to determine and explain the face validity of the instrument.

Content validity.   Content validity is similar to face validity, but it is somewhat more specific and systematic. The purpose of content validity is to determine if the instrument measures all parts of the concept or variable being measured. The researcher must classify or categorize all parts of the concept being measured and then determine if the measuring tool includes all components.

Criterion validity.   "Criterion validity assesses the accuracy of a new measurement procedure by comparing it with some criterion *assumed* to be valid."[7] A valid standard, however, must be found. There are two types of criterion validity based on different standards. *Concurrent validity* is determined by comparing a new tool that is proposed to measure a specific variable with a tool that measures the same variable and has already been determined to be valid. *Predictive validity* involves the ability of a measuring tool to predict something based on the results of the tool. If a measuring tool predicts that certain behaviors in an individual will occur and those behaviors do in fact occur at some later time, the tool is said to have predictive validity.

Construct validity.   Construct validity involves a much more complex procedure, usually involving statistical procedures. This type of validity is concerned with determining the interrelationships among the various constructs (components) of the concept being measured.

Reliability.   Reliability means that the instrument measures a variable consistently. For example, if a test is reliable, essentially the same results should be obtained for the same person over a period of time and in different situations. Seaman and Verhonick[8] identified three major concepts related to reliability: (1) stability, which determines how consistent the results of the test are over time; (2) internal homogeneity, which determines to what extent all of the items in the test measure the same characteristic; and (3) equivalence, which determines to what extent two different forms of a test will measure the same thing or two different researchers will observe or measure the same thing.

Utilizing Standardized Scales and Tests

The validity and reliability of the instruments used in a study are very important. If the researcher can locate a standardized scale or test to measure the variables needed to answer the research question, the quality of the research and the value of the findings will be enhanced. Several resources that will aid in the search for the right instrument are listed in the references.[9-11] While reviewing the literature, the beginning researcher should also be alert to instruments that have been developed and/or used by experienced nurse researchers. Contacting these authors for more information about their research, and specifically the instruments they have used, may be worth the effort. A letter or a telephone call with the request will often bring results because nurse authors/researchers are usually eager to share their expertise with novice researchers.

If a published standardized instrument is used, however, the nurse must usually purchase the specific number needed for the study because the instruments are copyrighted. If an instrument is published in a book or journal but is not standardized, written permission will need to be obtained from the publisher and/or author, and sometimes a fee will be required.

Instrumentation

Seaman and Verhonick defined instrumentation as "the construction and use of instruments in the observation, measurement, and analysis of data."[12] If an instrument cannot be found that can be used to collect the data needed to answer the research question, development of a new instrument may be necessary. The same considerations about validity and reliability need to be demonstrated when an instrument is constructed as when standardized tests and scales are chosen and used. Therefore, it is not recommended that the beginning researcher become involved in the development of new instruments unless there is adequate time and unless experienced nurse researchers are available for consultation. This does not mean that observation checklists, questionnaires, and interview guides should not be developed for descriptive and/or exploratory studies. In fact, the beginning researcher might want to start with such a study.

If an observation checklist, questionnaire, or interview guide is developed by the researcher, the development should include a small pilot study. The pilot study gives the researcher an opportunity to test out the instrument on a small group of subjects (five to ten or so, depending on the time available for development of the instrument) who meet the same criteria as those to be selected for the study. This process is essential if the instrument is a new one. The pilot study helps the researcher to determine if the instrument "works."

If the instrument is an observation guide, testing it out will determine if there are an adequate number of categories for the observed behaviors. If the instrument is a questionnaire to be completed by subjects, the pilot study will help the researcher to determine if the questions are clear and understood by the subjects. The pilot study data also help to determine if the type of responses made by the subjects can be summarized and categorized so that analysis and conclusions can be made from the data.

SELECTION OF SUBJECTS

If the study involves people in some way, the next step in the research process is the selection of subjects. The subjects are those people—patients, clients, other nurses, students—from whom the researcher needs to collect specific data to answer the research question. The researcher will need to decide:

- How many subjects are needed.
- Where they can be located.
- The criteria for their selection.
- Exactly how they will be selected.

The Number of Subjects

The number (n) of subjects to be used in the study will depend upon several factors, one of which is the methodological approach to be used. If an inductive approach with a nonstructured interview methodology is to be used, the researcher might want to limit the number of subjects to ten or so. If a deductive approach with a structured mailed questionnaire is to be used and quantitative statistical analysis of the data will be made, the lowest limit is about thirty. A greater number is always preferred, however, because of several factors. Sometimes the data obtained from several subjects may not be usable because of missing data. Or subjects may drop out of the study because they are discharged from the hospital or because they prefer not to continue to participate in the research. Summary, analysis, and conclusions also are less meaningful when the number of subjects is very small.

The number of subjects to be used will also depend upon the availability of subjects needed to answer the research question. For example, if the nurse wants to interview newly diagnosed diabetic children, ages six to ten, in a 200-bed children's hospital, there may be only one or two such patients admitted in a month. Therefore, it may take one year or more to identify and interview enough subjects, whose physician and parents approve of the child's participation in the research, to complete the study and obtain any kind of results.

The researcher's time commitment and financial resources also need to be considered when deciding on the number of subjects to be included in the study. A student may have a time limit of one or two semesters to complete a study. A staff nurse on a busy hospital unit may need to collect data outside of working hours. Equipment or supplies such as sphygmomanometers or videotapes may be needed. Even if equipment or supplies can be borrowed from the university or clinical agency, a limited number may be available. There are more exact and complex methods of determining *sample size* for the advanced researcher.

Where to Locate Subjects

Assuming that the nurse is planning to do a clinical nursing study, one or more clinical agencies will probably be chosen. The agency may be a hospital, outpatient clinic, home health agency, extended care facility, surgery outpatient center, or adult day care center. *Wherever there are patients and/or clients, there are potential subjects*. The final choice will depend upon the research question and whether or not the agency will allow the researcher to conduct the study in the agency.

Although nurses may want to conduct small studies in the agencies and units where they work, sometimes it is better to seek a different setting because of the possibility of researcher bias. This suggestion is especially true if some type of observation is the method used to collect data. Researchers may find it very difficult to be objective observers of patients and/or staff on the units where they work every day.

Another factor to consider is the type of subjects available in the agency. For example, choosing subjects in several small proprietary (for-profit) hospitals in suburban areas will bias the results if the research is intended to study the effect of prenatal care on length of labor. Patients should be selected from a variety of hospitals, including large public hospitals in the inner city. The assumption, whether correct or not, is that obstetrical patients in proprietary hospitals are more likely to have private physicians and, therefore, better prenatal care than obstetrical patients in large public hospitals in cities. A large teaching hospital associated with a medical school may more likely give approval and assistance with the study than a proprietary hospital with private patients. The selection of patients may still produce bias, however, if the patients in the hospital are primarily in the low-income category. A variety of agencies should be used if the results are to be generalized to a larger population.

Criteria for Selection

The nurse researcher must decide specific criteria for the selection of subjects needed for the study. For example, if the nurse plans to interview patients and speaks only the English language, one of the criteria for selection must be that the subjects are English speaking. There may be very few or multiple criteria. The criteria may be broad or specific. Sample types of criteria that might be used in the selection of subjects are:

- Age (for example, between 13 and 19 *or* 85 and over)
- Medical diagnosis and/or type of surgery (for example, elective orthopedic surgery)
- Number of days postoperative or postdelivery (for example, first 24 hours or third day)
- Type of medications being taken (for example, no narcotics or tranquilizers being taken during the period of the study)

These criteria, of course, will depend upon the research problem/question, and specific criteria are needed to determine the specific selection of subjects.

Method of Selection

The most important factor in the selection of subjects is the specific method of selection. Four major kinds of sampling techniques that the beginning researcher may decide to use are:

- Sample of convenience
- Quota sample

- Simple random sample
- Stratified random sample

Sample of Convenience.   A sample of convenience, sometimes called an *accidental sample,* simply means choosing those subjects who are conveniently available. Specific criteria for selection are utilized, but there is no other specific methodology used in the selection. If the research is a small descriptive or exploratory study, a sample of convenience may be used. If there are a limited number of subjects available who meet the criteria, a convenience sample may be the only one possible. However, if there are only a few subjects who meet the criteria for selection, the researcher must ask whether or not the research question is worth the time and effort to study. A sample of convenience is a type of nonprobability sampling that does not allow for generalization to a larger population because it does not represent that population and is, therefore, less effective.

Quota Sample.   Another type of nonprobability sampling is the quota sample. This type of sample is different from the sample of convenience in that a specific number or percentage of subjects are selected from different groups of subjects in order to obtain a more representative sample.

Simple Random Sample.   A random sample is a type of probability sampling in which every subject in a particular population group has the same chance of being chosen; thus, the sample represents the total population. If the study uses a deductive approach and hypotheses are to be tested by statistical means (see Chapter 7), a random sample is usually needed. Many statistical tools are based on the premise that a random sample was utilized in the selection of subjects.

The researcher first chooses the specific criteria for selection, as discussed previously. All individuals who meet these criteria are labeled as the *universe.* Because it is impossible and not necessary to study the universe (all people who meet the criteria), a specific portion of the universe, a *population*, is chosen. The population may consist of all people who meet the selected criteria in a specific location (such as county, state, city, or hospital). The choice of specific population will depend upon some of the other factors of selection previously discussed, such as number of subjects, time commitment of the researcher, and financial resources available.

After the population has been chosen, a *random sample* is chosen from that population. The random sample represents the population that represents the universe. The results that are analyzed from the data collected from the random sample, therefore, can be *generalized* (if proper statistical methodology was used) to the total population. Because specific results occurred in one small group of subjects, it can be said that *the same could have occurred in the total population because the sample came from that population*. Such a technique, therefore, makes the findings more applicable in a wider variety of settings (see Figure 6–1). The concept of generalizability is very important in research. If the results of a study cannot be generalized to a larger population than the specific sample studied, the time, energy, and resources utilized for the study can be questioned because of the limited applicability of the findings.

The technique of choosing a random sample usually involves the use of a table of random numbers that has been prepared by statisticians to assure that there is no rationale

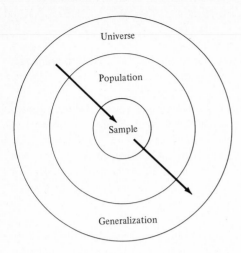

FIGURE 6–1
Comparison of universe, population, and sample.

for the numbering system. A table of random numbers can be found in the appendix of any basic statistics textbook. The researcher simply selects one of the numbers (1, 2, or 3 digits depending upon the size of the sample desired) and counts up or down until the number of subjects desired are chosen. The population will have previously been numbered (for example from one to ninety-nine). If twenty subjects are desired, the first twenty numbers on the table of random numbers will comprise the random sample. Choosing every fifth number in a list or drawing numbers out of a container does not provide a random sample because every number does not have an equal chance of being chosen. Once a number is selected and deleted, the chance for the other numbers to be chosen increases because there are fewer numbers from which to select.

Stratified Random Sample.   Another type of probability sampling is the stratified random sample, which means that several different kinds of populations are chosen in order to broaden the generalizability of the random sample. Population groups may be chosen on the basis of:

- Sex
- Geographical location
- Educational background
- Income

A random sample will then be chosen from each of these population groups to become the total sample. A stratified random sample is more likely to be used in major studies involving large population groups than in small studies in specific clinical settings.

APPROVALS NEEDED TO CONDUCT THE RESEARCH

Although the research plan is well under way and the method of data collection and sampling decided, there is another important phase of research before the collection of data can begin. Because of the nature of nursing research, that is, the involvement of patients, clients, and other individuals in clinical settings, the nurse researcher will need to obtain approval from several sources.

Nursing students will need to obtain approval from their teachers, advisers, and/or project directors—whoever is responsible for assisting with the research study. A department committee on research will usually also need to approve the research proposal. Practicing nurses will need to obtain approval from their immediate superiors, perhaps a head nurse or supervisor. Both the student and the agency nurse will need approval from the clinical agency research committee. Details for obtaining these approvals will be discussed in Chapter 12.

Informed Consent Procedures

Nurses are probably quite familiar with the concept of informed consent because of the requirement in most agencies that all patients must sign a consent form to give permission for surgery, certain diagnostic procedures, and specific types of medical treatment. The signature of the patient on the consent form implies that he or she has been informed about what the procedure involves as well as the possible benefits and risks resulting from it. It is the physician's responsibility to explain the medical treatment to the patient, although the nurses ask patients if they understand the explanation and then witness the patients' signatures on the consent forms.

Informed consent is required in any research project that involves human subjects, whether these subjects are patients, clients, family, friends, colleagues, or students.

Reasons for Informed Consent.   The concept of informed consent is one that implies that all individuals have human worth and dignity, that they have control over their own bodies, and that they should not be subjected to any kind of research that could harm them. There were individuals in the 1930s and 1940s who were involved in research studies without their consent and sometimes knowledge. Research studies involving prisoners, mentally retarded children and adults in institutions, and military personnel were conducted, in some cases with severely detrimental results to the individuals involved.

Current guidelines used for the protection of human subjects in research have their origins in the Nuremberg Code, which resulted from experiments on prisoners of war without their consent during World War II; the Declaration of Helsinki (1964 and revised in 1975), which provided physicians with guidelines in biomedical research, and the United States Department of Health, Education, and Welfare (now the Department of Health and Human Services),[13] which has described in the Federal Register[14] regulations on informed consent.

Guidelines.   Every institution that receives federal funds of some kind (this includes almost all health care institutions in one way or another) must follow federal regulations for informed consent in their institutions. The federal regulations have become less stringent in recent years, especially if the research does not involve a physical element. However, because informed consent is an important ethical issue for the protection of the welfare of human subjects, specific informed consent procedures continue to be vital in conducting research involving human subjects.

The Informed Consent Form. When the researcher prepares the research proposal (see Chapter 9), informed consent procedures must be included in the proposal. A university and/or clinical agency committee on research will review the proposal for the proper informed consent procedures (see sample form in Appendix C). These procedures will involve the preparation of an *informed consent form* of some type. There is no standard format for this form, although a specific agency may require its own. The form should include the following components:

- Brief explanation of the purpose and procedures of the research
- Description of the possible benefits, discomforts, and risks to the subject
- Provisions for anonymity
- Statement that participation is completely voluntary and that the subject is free to withdraw at any time
- Explanation about from whom and where the subject can ask questions and receive final results of the study[15]
- The date and signatures of the subject, the researcher, and an objective witness

Two examples of informed consent forms are included in Appendices D and E. One is an example of a form required by a clinical agency. The other one is a general form suggested by a university committee. A short form is usually preferred because it seems to be more acceptable to subjects.

Tape-recorded interviews may include verbal agreement by the subject at the beginning of the interview. Questionnaires sent by mail and telephone interviews do not have to have a signed informed consent form. However, the researcher should explain in the cover letter of the questionnaire the components listed earlier. A statement can then be used such as: "Completion of this questionnaire implies informed consent." A similar process can be used for telephone interviews with the statement such as: "Responding to these questions implies informed consent." Of course, subjects can stop the interview anytime they want to simply by hanging up the phone.

Extenuating circumstances. If the subject is under legal age (usually 21), one or both of the parents or a legal guardian must sign the informed consent form. If the subject is anesthetized, unconscious for any reason, confused, or mentally disturbed, the nearest family member or a legal guardian must sign the form. Age is no barrier to research that may benefit others; however, some interpretations imply that ethically subjects should not participate in any research unless they can give their own consent.[16]

If the subject cannot read or write, the contents of the form should be read to the subject and a written symbol X obtained. In this instance, the signature of at least one witness should also be obtained. Sometimes subjects, especially the elderly, are reluctant to sign their names on the consent forms even though they agree verbally to participate in the research. Research on the elderly, for example, is especially needed because of the many problems of the increasing older population. However, strict informed consent is sometimes difficult to obtain, especially in the old-old (over 85) age group and the institutionalized.[17] A careful and clear explanation of the need for a signature may convince elderly subjects to sign. If not, verbal agreement with the signature of a witness can be used. The researcher must remember that potential subjects have the right to refuse to participate and they must not be pressured to do so.

Obtaining the Approvals

All of the approvals required and the informed consent procedures may seem like obstacles to the beginning researcher. However, these steps are essential before the collection of data can begin. The nurse researcher must be persistent and accept this phase as one of the rigorous requirements of research. The clinical agency staff and subjects often understand the research better because of these approval procedures, however, and thus result in increased cooperation and support as the collection of data proceeds.

SUMMARY

The collection of data is often the major and most interesting part of the research study. The data to be collected must be able to answer the research question(s). The major methods of data collection are observation, questionnaires, interviews, physical data, records and reports, standardized scales and tests, and selection or construction of a new instrument. There are several advantages and disadvantages to each approach. The beginning researcher may need to consult with an experienced researcher to determine which method is the most appropriate to study the specific research problem.

The selection of subjects is another important part of data collection procedures. The researcher will need to decide: (1) how many subjects are needed, (2) where they can be located, (3) the criteria for their selection, and (4) exactly how they will be selected. Three major types of subject samples are: (1) convenience (or accidental) sample, (2) random sample, and (3) stratified random sample.

Before the process of data collection can begin, the researcher will need to obtain approval for the study from several individuals and/or groups. The student will need approval from a teacher and/or project adviser and perhaps a university or college research committee. Clinical agency nurses will need approval from their immediate superiors. Both will need approval of the research committee in the clinical agency where the study is to be conducted. The researcher must also follow informed consent procedures of the institutions involved if human subjects are used in the study. These approval procedures may sometimes seem like obstacles to implementing a research study in a clinical setting, but they are necessary and often result in increased cooperation and support by the agency personnel. Chapter 12 expands on the implementation of research in a clinical setting.

QUESTIONS FOR STUDY AND DISCUSSION

   1 What is the primary purpose of data collection?
   2 Name seven methods of collecting data.

3 Discuss the advantages and disadvantages of the major methods of data collection.

4 Discuss the importance of instrument validity and reliability.

5 List and define five types of validity.

6 What is the lower limit for number of subjects in a deductive study utilizing statistical analysis?

7 List and discuss the three types of sampling.

8 Discuss the rationale for informed consent procedures in research.

9 Name six components that should be included in the informed consent form.

10 How should the researcher obtain informed consent from a subject who is blind? One who is a child? One who is confused?

REFERENCES

1 Pamela J. Brink, and Marilyn J. Wood, *Basic Steps in Planning Nursing Research,* Duxbury Press, North Scituate, Massachusetts, 1978, p. 105.

2 Brink and Wood, ibid., pp. 90–91.

3 Denise F. Polit, and Bernadette P. Hungler, *Nursing Research,* Lippincott, Philadelphia, 1983, p. 317.

4 Diane K. Dressler, Carol Smejkal, and Mary Lee Ruffolo, "A Comparison of Oral and Rectal Temperature Measurement on Patients Receiving Oxygen by Mask," *Nursing Research,* vol. 32, no. 6, 1983, pp. 373–375.

5 Nancy C. Baker et al., "The Effect of Type of Thermometer and Length of Time Inserted on Oral Temperature Measurements of Afebrile Subjects," *Nursing Research,* vol. 33, no. 2, 1984, pp. 109–111.

6 Michael H. Walizer, and Paul L. Wienir, *Research Methods and Analysis,* Harper & Row, New York, 1978, pp. 409–410.

7 Walizer and Wienir, ibid., p. 411.

8 Catherine H. C. Seaman, and Phyllis J. Verhonick, *Research Methods,* 2d ed., Appleton-Century-Crofts, Norwalk, Connecticut, 1982, pp. 241–242.

9 Mary Jane Ward, and Carol A. Lindeman, *Instruments for Measuring Nursing Practice and Other Health Care Variables,* Western Interstate Commission for Higher Education, Boulder, Colorado, 1978.

10 Mary Jane Ward, and Mark E. Fetter, *Instruments for Use in Nursing Education Research,* Western Interstate Commission for Higher Education, Boulder, Colorado, 1979.

11 James V. Mitchell, Jr. (ed.), *Tests in Print III,* University of Nebraska Press, Lincoln, 1983.

12 Seaman and Verhonick, op. cit., p. 192.

13 Robert M. Veatch, *Case Studies in Medical Ethics,* Harvard University Press, Cambridge, Massachusetts, 1977, pp. 357–367.

14 Federal Register, 45 CFR 46, January 26, 1981.

15 Veatch, op. cit., p. 364

16 Veatch, op. cit., p. 297.

17 Susanne S. Robb, "Beware the 'Informed' Consent," (editorial), *Nursing Research,* vol. 32, no. 3, 1983, p. 132.

BIBLIOGRAPHY

Brink, Pamela J., and Marilyn J. Wood, *Basic Steps in Planning Nursing Research,* Duxbury Press, North Scituate, Massachusetts, 1978.

Holm, Karyn, "Single Subject Research," *Nursing Research,* vol. 32, no. 4, 1983, pp. 253–255.

Kelly, Kathleen, and Eleanor McClelland, "Signed Consent: Protection or Constraint?", *Nursing Outlook,* vol. 27, no. 1, 1979, pp. 40–42.

May, Katharyn Antle, "The Nurse as Researcher: Impediment to Informed Consent?", *Nursing Outlook,* vol. 27, no. 1, 1979, pp. 36–39.

Polit, Denise F., and Bernadette P. Hungler, *Nursing Research,* Lippincott, Philadelphia, 1983.

Seaman, Catherine H. C., and Phyllis J. Verhonick, *Research Methods,* 2d ed., Appleton-Century-Crofts, Norwalk, Connecticut, 1982.

CHAPTER 7

ANALYSIS OF DATA

Analysis of quantitative data usually occurs after the final completion of data collection, unless analysis of early pilot study data is needed to refine the design or instruments used. However, analysis of qualitative data in an inductive study using the grounded theory approach is an ongoing process with summary at the completion of the study. As discussed in Chapter 6, the researcher should determine the method(s) of data analysis before beginning to collect data. Otherwise, data may be collected that is difficult, if not impossible, to analyze in any way. The method of data analysis will depend upon the research design and will be described in this chapter.

After the data have been collected, the researcher must analyze, or make sense out of, the data so that a summary or conclusion can be drawn from the findings. Methods of analyzing the data range from the very simple to multiple complex statistical procedures. This chapter will introduce the beginning researcher to several of the most basic methods of analysis. If it was not required in the basic nursing program, an introductory course in elementary statistics is highly recommended for all nurses who wish to pursue research in the practice setting and/or graduate school. If a statistics course is not taught in the nursing curriculum, a beginning course can usually be found in the departments of mathematics, psychology, sociology, education, and/or business of most universities or colleges.

LEVELS OF MEASUREMENT

Before statistical procedures can be discussed, it is necessary to review the levels or types of measurement because they will be referred to later in the chapter. The major levels of measurement are:

- Discrete
  Nominal
  Ordinal
- Continuous
  Interval
  Ratio

Discrete Measurement

Discrete measurement means that the data is categorical and cannot be assigned specific numerical values. Nominal and ordinal variables are types of discrete measurement.

Nominal Measurement.   Nominal measurement is used primarily to assign variable values to mutually exclusive, nonnumerical categories. These categories do not represent quantities of a variable, but merely distinguish between groups. Examples of types of observations or factors that require nominal measurement are sex, religion, occupation, and geographical location. One can describe the quantity of subjects who are of a specific religion, but a religion itself cannot be quantified.

Ordinal Measurement.   Ordinal measurement is used to measure levels of a category or characteristic. These levels can be ranked or ordered, but they are non-numerical, since distance between ranks cannot be measured. Therefore, ratios cannot be established for ordinal data and neither can an absolute zero point be determined. For example, a specific characteristic can be placed in a *high* or *low* category, but it is not known how much higher high is than low. Ordinal measurement provides order among several categories.

Continuous Measurement

Continuous measurement means that data points can be assigned a numeric value. Examples of continuous measurement are interval and ratio measurements.

Interval Measurement.   When interval measurement is used, data points are measured in equidistant quantitative values of a specific factor or characteristic. Vital signs, for example, illustrate interval measurement because all four of them (temperature, pulse, respiration, and blood pressure) can be measured in successive numbers. However, interval measures have no true, absolute zero point. Thus, the meaning associated with a given value, while perhaps having became widely known and accepted, was probably originally a somewhat arbitrary designation.

Ratio Measurement.   Ratio measurement is very similar to interval measurement except that ratio measurement involves the use of a true absolute zero. Height and weight are examples of ratio variables. Each of these has a true zero in that it is meaningful to speak of zero weight or, in essence, weightlessness. This differs from interval measurements such as temperature because there is no real sense of absence of temperature.

USE OF STATISTICS

Statistical techniques are those scientific procedures that help the researcher to collect, organize, summarize, and analyze information in some way.[1] Some nurses feel that they are not knowledgeable in the field of mathematics. Although highly related, statistical techniques are, in a sense, really different from mathematics in the way math is thought about by many people.

The most important thing to learn about statistics is that the right technique, procedure, or formula must be selected and used based on the research purpose and/or hypotheses and the type of data collected. Consultation with someone who is knowledgeable about statistics and the use of statistical computer packages make this phase of the research process much less complicated for the beginning nurse researcher than one might think. It is essential to consult with a statistician *before* beginning the research project. This process may prevent the researcher from ending up with useless data. A knowledgeable researcher can save the beginning researcher many disappointments and wasted hours.

A list of the most common abbreviations and symbols used in analyzing statistical data, together with brief definitions of each, will be found in Table 7–1. These terms and symbols will be especially useful to know when reading research literature.

TYPES OF STATISTICS

The two major categories of statistics to be presented in this chapter are *descriptive* and *inferential*.

Descriptive Statistics

Descriptive statistics includes those procedures or techniques that help to categorize, summarize, describe, and give evident meaning to a set or group of things. For example, note the raw data in Table 7–2. What are these numbers and what do they mean? Are they ages? Are they scores on a test? How does one number relate to any one or all of the other numbers? The numbers alone mean nothing.

Various types of simple descriptive statistics can be utilized to organize these types of data to give them meaning. Some of the statistical techniques which can be used to describe the data in Table 7–2 (page 101) are:

- Number (n)
- Range (R)
- Mean (M, Mn or $\overline{X}$)
- Median (Md)

TABLE 7–1

COMMON ABBREVIATIONS AND SYMBOLS USED IN ANALYZING STATISTICAL DATA

Abbreviation or Symbol	Meaning	Definition
N	Number	Population size
n	Number	Sample size
X	Individual data points or observations	Individual raw numbers
R	Range	Largest data point (or observation) minus smallest data point
Σ	Summa	Sum or total of all the data points
M or Mn or $\bar{X}$	Mean of the sample	Sum or total of all data points divided by the number of observations in the sample.
μ	Mean of the population	
Md	Median	Middle number in a set of numbers
Mo	Mode	Most common number occurring in a set of numbers.
t-test	t-test	Statistical test used to determine if there is a significant difference between the means of two sets of observations
r	Correlation	Test to determine whether changes in the value of one variable occur consistently with a systematic change in values of another variable
df	Degrees of freedom	Number of terms that are measured
H_1	Research hypothesis #1	What the researcher expects to occur
Ho	Null hypothesis	Statement of no observable effect in an experiment due to manipulation of the variables being measured.

- Mode (Mo)
- Frequency distribution (fd)
- Percentage (%)
- Standard deviation (S or s)

Number (n).   The first descriptive statistic is simply the total number. Looking at the numbers in Table 7–2, it can be seen that there are five rows of six numbers each, for a total n of *30* in this sample. There are 30 numbers, which is more information known

TABLE 7–1 (continued)
COMMON ABBREVIATIONS AND SYMBOLS USED IN ANALYZING STATISTICAL DATA

Abbreviation or Symbol	Meaning	Definition
$p \leqslant 0.05$	Probability is that the statistical level of significance is equal to or less than 0.05.	Null hypothesis is rejected if the level of significance is equal to or less than 0.05.
fd	Frequency distribution	Graph portraying the numbers of data points grouped into each interval or category
%	Percentage	Proportion of 100
S or s	Standard deviation of the sample.	Average of all of the deviations from the mean
σ	Standard deviation of the population.	
$>$	Greater than	Same
$<$	Less than	Same
$\sqrt{}$	Square root	Number for which the given number is the square
χ^2	Chi square	Statistical test used to determine if there is a significant difference between the frequency of occurrences in categories of observations (data)

about the data in Table 7–2 than before the numbers were counted. The total n of subjects, scores, vital signs, or whatever type of data is available or collected is the first place to start.

Range (R). The range is determined by subtracting the smallest number from the largest number. From looking at Table 7–2, it is evident that the largest number is 96 and the smallest number is 6. Therefore, the range is determined as follows:

$$R = 96 - 6$$
$$R = 90$$

This additional descriptive technique shows that the range is rather large for an n of 30, so that there is much difference between the highest and lowest numbers.

Mean (Mn or $\overline{X}$). The mean is simply the arithmetic average and is determined by adding all of the individual numbers and dividing by the total number in the sample as follows:

$$\overline{X} = \frac{\Sigma X}{n}$$

TABLE 7–2
A SAMPLE OF NUMBERS AS RAW DATA

18	55	13	38	57
66	22	30	24	87
50	89	79	90	28
6	38	68	38	69
42	77	48	59	44
78	33	15	96	43

where Σ is the summation sign, X represents each individual number, and n equals the total number of observations in the sample.

$$\Sigma X = (18 + 55 + 13 \ldots 96 + 43)$$
$$\bar{X} = 1500 \div 30$$
$$\bar{X} = 50$$

The mean, therefore, is 50, which provides additional descriptive information about the numbers in Table 7–2. The larger the total number of numbers, the more accurate the true mean. The mean, however, provides no information about the range or dispersion of the observations. The range may be relatively large (for example, 90) or small (for example, 5). The observations may be uniformly distributed across the range or heavily clustered at one end.

Median (Md). The median is the middle number in a group of numbers. In order to determine the median, it is necessary to rearrange all of the numbers from the highest to the lowest (or vice versa) as shown in Table 7–3. One could count down (or up) to the middle number to find the median. However, if the n is an even number, as is the case in Table 7–3, there is no obvious middle number because there are 15 numbers at the top and 15 numbers at the bottom. Therefore, the median will fall between the two middle numbers. The two middle numbers are added together and divided by 2, as shown in Table 7–3, to find the median of 46. It should be noted that the median (46) is close to but less than the mean (50). The median is not affected by extremely high or low scores like the mean, which is an average score.

Mode (Mo). The mode is the most frequently occurring number. The mode is very easy to determine, therefore, by noting which number occurs most often in the sample. The mode in the numbers in Table 7–3 is 38 because this number occurs three times. In some sets of numbers there may be several modes (several numbers occurring the same number of times) or no mode (if no one number occurs more than one time). The mode, therefore, although easily determined by observation as a rough estimate of the average, is not very useful.

TABLE 7–3
REARRANGEMENT OF NUMBERS IN TABLE 7–2 AND CALCULATION OF MEDIAN, MODE, AND MEAN

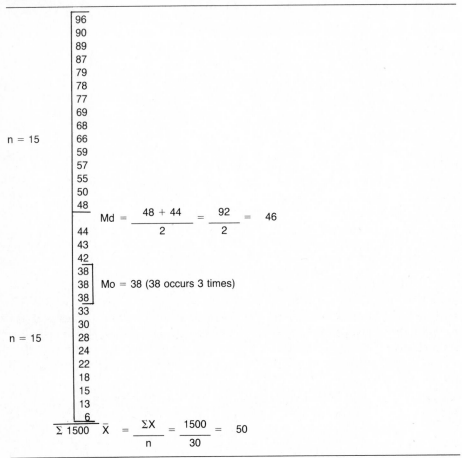

Frequency Distribution (fd). If there were more than a few numbers to organize and summarize, however, it would be tedious and unnecessary to list all of the numbers separately, as shown in Table 7–3. Instead, a frequency distribution can be made to organize a large group of numbers, especially if some of the same numbers occur frequently. First, frequency *intervals* are determined by the researcher, depending on the range and total numbers (for example, intervals of 5, 10, 15, 20, or so). Then a count is taken of the number of observations falling into each interval. Table 7–4 shows a frequency distribution with intervals of 10. Each interval must be equal and mutually exclusive; that is, numerical boundaries of intervals must not overlap. Overlapping boundaries make it impossible to determine to which category borderline observations should be assigned. The frequency distribution in Table 7–4 shows that the observations

TABLE 7–4
FREQUENCY DISTRIBUTION AND PERCENTAGE

Intervals	Frequency	Number
90–99	11	2
80–89	11	2
70–79	111	3
60–69	111	3
50–59	1111	4
40–49	1111	4
30–39	11111	5
20–29	111	3
10–19	111	3
*0– 9	1	1

$N = \dfrac{14}{30} = 46.7\%$ (50 or above)

$N = \dfrac{9}{30} = 30\%$ (between 30 and 49)

$N = \dfrac{16}{30} = 53.3\%$ (49 or below)

*Note that each interval is 10.

are evenly distributed with the heaviest concentration of observations (9) between 30 and 49.

Percentage (%).   Percentage is the rate or proportion of 100 represented by some variable or set of data points. This simple calculation has meaning and can be used by the beginning researcher who cannot or prefers not to use detailed statistical procedures. The percentage is often used in simple descriptive studies and in inductive exploratory field studies where there is analysis of descriptive data obtained, for example, from observation, open-ended interviews, or questionnaires.

The percentage is calculated by dividing any part of the whole by the whole. For example, it can be seen in Table 7–4 that 14 (14/30 or 46.7%) of the numbers fall in the area from 50 to 100 and 16 (16/30 or 53.3%) of the numbers from 0 to 49. Therefore, there are more numbers below 50 than at 50 or above. Also, it can be seen that 9 (30%) of the numbers fall between 30 and 49, which means that a greater percentage of numbers fall in those two combined intervals than in any of the other two combined intervals.

If the data are in raw numbers and no major statistical procedures are going to be used, percentages should be used. Whenever referring to a raw number, the percentage should also be given. It is not sufficient to give the raw number *or* the percentage, but both together will give more complete information. See an example of the use of both in the pie graph in Figure 7–1.

Percentage should be differentiated from percentile rank. Percentile rank is the point below which a certain percentage of the numbers fall. For example, a number at the sixtieth percentile means that there are 60 numbers below that number in a group of numbers. Percentiles are often used in reporting test scores (for example, National League for Nursing Achievement Test scores), but are not used as often in classifying descriptive data in research. It is important that these two terms (percentages and percentile) be used correctly.

Standard Deviations (S). The standard deviation is the average of the deviations of all of the numbers from the mean. The standard deviation helps to determine the degree of error of the mean of a set of numbers.[2] This statistic is slightly more difficult to determine than the mean; however, calculation begins with the mean and can be performed easily by using the formula below and following the sample shown in Table 7–5.

$$S = \sqrt{\frac{\Sigma x^2}{n}}$$

(standard deviation = the square root of the sum of the deviations from the mean squared divided by the total number)

Measures of Central Tendency. Besides providing specific methods to describe a set of numbers, several of the procedures just discussed generate statistics that can be used to be representative of the total group of numbers. The mean, median, mode, standard deviation, and frequency distribution all are measures of central tendency of a group of numbers. That is, these numbers give various estimates that describe the center of the set of numbers. A summary of the descriptive statistical procedures calculated for the raw numbers in Table 7–2 is listed in Table 7–6. Much more information is now known about the numbers in Table 7–2 than was possible when simply looking at the raw numbers.

Use of Graphs to Present Descriptive Statistics. Descriptive statistics can be summarized and illustrated in a graph of some type. The most common types of graphs used are the: (1) histogram, (2) polygon, (3) bar graph, and (4) pie graph. A sample of each of these graphs is shown in Figure 7–1. Note that frequency distributions can be graphically illustrated on a histogram or frequency polygon. Percentages are quite often shown on a bar graph or pie graph.

All of the graphs in Figure 7–1 depict the data originally presented in Table 7–2. Which of the four graphs is the most descriptive? Which one would be most useful in presenting the data? Researchers can decide which method would best illustrate their own descriptive data. It often helps to try several methods before deciding which one to use. Additional suggestions on how to use and label graphs in an oral presentation and written report are given in Chapter 9.

Inferential Statistics

Inferential statistics refers to those statistical procedures and/or formulas that are used to make specific inferences, generalizations, and/or conclusions from the data. Several of the simpler techniques will be presented that the beginning researcher may want to use. While access to a computer will make utilization of these procedures very simple and easy, the inferential statistical procedures presented in this chapter can be performed with a hand calculator if desired (especially if the n is relatively small). Before discussing the specific statistical tests listed above, there are several basic concepts that must be presented because they are used when discussing these tests. These concepts include: (1) variables, (2) null hypotheses, and (3) levels of significance.

TABLE 7-5
CALCULATION OF STANDARD DEVIATION

X (individual numbers)	χ (deviation of each number from the mean)	χ^2 (each deviation squared)
96	(−50) = 46 (X46) =	2116
90	40	1600
89	39	1521
87	37	1369
79	29	841
78	28	784
77	27	729
69	19	361
68	18	324
66	16	256
59	9	81
57	7	49
55	5	25
50	0	0
48	−2 (−X− = +)	4
44	−6	36
43	−7	49
42	−8	64
38	−12	144
38	−12	144
38	−12	144
33	−17	289
30	−20	400
28	−22	484
24	−26	676
22	−28	784
18	−32	1024
15	−35	1225
13	−37	1369
6	−44	1936
$\Sigma X = 1500$ $n = 30$		$\Sigma\chi^2 = 18828$

$$\bar{X} = \frac{\Sigma X}{n} \qquad\qquad S = \sqrt{\frac{\Sigma\chi^2}{n}}$$

$$\bar{X} = \frac{1500}{30} \qquad\qquad S = \sqrt{\frac{18828}{30}}$$

$$\bar{X} = 50 \qquad\qquad S = \sqrt{627.6}$$

$$S = 25.05$$

TABLE 7–6
DESCRIPTIVE STATISTICS SUMMARIZED FOR NUMBERS IN TABLE 7–2

Statistic	Number
n	30
R	90
$\bar{X}$	50
Md	46
Mo	38
fd	30 − 49 = 9 = 30%
S	25.05

FIGURE 7–1
Samples of the histogram, frequency polygon, bar graph, and pie graph.

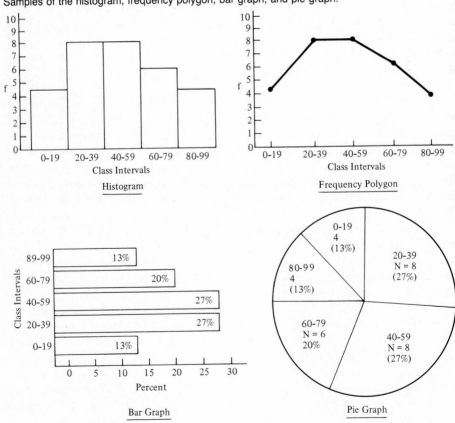

Note that two class intervals have been combined to make five classes rather than ten, as shown in Table 7-4.

Variable. A variable is a characteristic that changes or can be manipulated experimentally with respect to its assigned value over time or from person to person. Variables may be *qualitative* (descriptive, such as the appearance of the skin) or quantitative (measurable, such as the temperature). An *independent* variable is something that influences or acts on other variables, while a *dependent* variable is something that is acted upon. For example, smoking (independent variable) affects (constricts) blood vessels (dependent variable). There may be numerous independent or dependent variables, however, and these variables must be differentiated when the researcher is attempting to discover or show a relationship among them. Being aware of and controlling all of the extraneous variables that could affect the results of the study is a major problem in doing research in a clinical setting.

Null Hypothesis. The null hypothesis was defined in Chapter 3. The null hypothesis may sound strange because it is stated in the negative form. For example, the following is stated as a null hypothesis: There will be no significant difference between the total hours of sleep from 9 PM to 7 AM for hospitalized children ages 4 to 7 who do and do not have at least one parent stay in the room with them. The *null hypothesis* seems awkward and may not be stated as such, but it is always implied if a statistical test is used to draw inferences from an experiment. The *research hypothesis* may state that hospitalized children ages 4 to 7 sleep just as well without one of their parents present as with one of them present.

Levels of Significance. In the discussion of descriptive statistics, the use of percentages was discussed. If 60 percent of the subjects in a specific study answered a question one way and 40 percent of the subjects in the same study answered the same question in a different way, the researcher can state that a *higher* percentage of subjects answered one way than another. However, using percentages, the researcher cannot state that 60 percent is *significantly* higher than 40 percent or that there is even a significant difference between 60 percent and 40 percent, although there *appears* to be a difference. These differences may have occurred by chance.

In inferential statistics data collected from a sample of subjects (who have been selected from a larger population) are used to make inferences or generalizations about the larger population from the sample. It is extremely important, therefore, that the sample be randomly selected (as discussed in Chapter 6) so that it is representative of the population as a whole and generalizations can be made.

Levels of significance indicate the probability that the results of the study would have occurred by chance; that is, due to random error rather than induced by a specific variable being tested and/or measured. This concept is important to understand when using inferential statistics in a research study. It is also necessary to understand the meaning of levels of significance when reading and evaluating published research reports as discussed in Chapter 8. When the statistical analysis of the data has been determined to be significant, this means that the researcher "has *rejected* the null hypothesis in favor of the research hypothesis."[3]

The minimum level of significance is considered by popular wisdom to be 0.05, although levels of 0.025, 0.01, 0.005, or even 0.0005 are sometimes required and obtained. A 0.05 level of significance means that no more than 5 times out of 100 (5 percent of the time) would the sample results have occurred by chance. When the null hypothesis is rejected at the 0.05 level of significance, it is written as $p \leq 0.05$. The researcher decides what level of significance will be required for a particular study at the beginning of the study. Levels of 0.01 or better may be required for a very important study of a new drug where the chance for error must be minimal. However, a level of 0.05 is satisfactory for most research.

Sometimes errors can be made such as rejecting or failing to reject the null hypothesis when the opposite is true. A Type I error means that the null hypothesis is rejected and the research hypothesis is accepted in error. If the null hypothesis fails to be rejected when it should have been rejected and the research hypothesis is rejected, a Type II error has occurred.

Statistical Tests. Some of the statistical tests which might be used by beginning researchers in order to make specific inferences from their data are the:

- t-test
  One-tailed
  Two-tailed
- Simple analysis of variance
- Chi square
- Correlation
  Rank-order method of correlation
  Pearson-product moment method of correlation

The t-test. If the researcher wants to compare the means of *two* groups of interval or ratio level data (for example, specific numbers or measurements), the t-test can be used as long as the two sets of data points are independent of each other. The t-test is used to determine if there is a *significant difference* between the means of two sets of numbers. The two-tailed t-test is most often used if the researcher does not need to know the direction of the difference between the means. The one-tailed t-test is used to determine the direction between two means. The t-test is a popular, powerful test that is widely used, especially when the number of subjects is relatively small (for example, thirty in each group). If the total number of the sample is smaller than that, a nonparametric procedure, such as chi square, should be used. If the t-test is used, it is assumed that the dependent variable is normally distributed in the two groups and that the standard deviations are very similar. If the n is equal in both groups, these assumptions are not as important.

The formula for the two-tailed t-test with an example from simulated data is shown in Table 7–7. The ns, means, and standard deviations have already been determined from the raw data (which is not shown).

After determining the total number (n), mean ($\overline{X}$), and standard deviation (S) for each of the two groups of numbers to be compared, the t-statistic can be calculated by following the sample in Table 7–7. After the degrees of freedom are determined, as shown in Table 7–7, the researcher will determine if the means are statistically different

TABLE 7–7
FORMULA AND CALCULATION OF A t-TEST SCORE

$$t = \frac{\bar{X}_1 - \bar{X}_2}{S\bar{X}_1 - \bar{X}_2}$$

where: $\bar{X}_1$ = the mean of the observations from sample 1
$\bar{X}_2$ = the mean of the observations from sample 2
$S\bar{X}_1$ = the standard error of the mean for sample 1
$S\bar{X}_2$ = the standard error of the mean for sample 2

$n = 36$ $\bar{X}_1 = 60$ $S_1 = 4.0$

$n = 36$ $\bar{X}_2 = 50$ $S_2 = 5.0$

$$S\bar{X}_1 = \frac{S_1}{\sqrt{n}} \qquad S\bar{X}_2 = \frac{S_2}{\sqrt{n}}$$

$$S\bar{X}_1 = \frac{4.0}{\sqrt{36}} \qquad S\bar{X}_2 = \frac{5.0}{\sqrt{36}}$$

$$S\bar{X}_1 = \frac{4.0}{\sqrt{6}} \qquad S\bar{X}_2 = \frac{5.0}{6}$$

$$S\bar{X}_1 = .67 \qquad S\bar{X}_2 = 0.83$$

$$S\bar{X}_1 - \bar{X}_2 = \sqrt{S\bar{X}_1^2 + S\bar{X}_2^2}$$

$$S\bar{X}_1 - \bar{X}_2 = \sqrt{0.67^2 + 0.83^2}$$

$$SX_1 - \bar{X}_2 = \sqrt{0.4489 + 0.6589}$$

$$SX_1 - \bar{X}_2 = \sqrt{1.1078}$$

$$SX_1 - \bar{X}_2 = 1.05$$

$$t = \frac{60 - 50}{1.05}$$

$$t = \frac{10}{1.05}$$

$$t = 9.52$$

$df = (N_1 - 1) + (N_2 = 1)$
(Formula for determining the degrees of freedom for the t-statistic)
$df = (36 - 1) + (36 - 1)$
$df = (35) + (35)$
$df = 70$

EXPLANATION:
1. The null hypothesis is stated as follows:
   Ho: There is *no* statistical difference between the means of samples 1 and 2.

2. The t- test statistic is $t = \dfrac{\bar{X}_1 - \bar{X}_2}{S\bar{X}_1 - S\bar{X}_2}$

TABLE 7–7 (continued)
FORMULA AND CALCULATION OF A t-TEST SCORE

3. The critical t-value for 0.05 is 1.980* and the degrees of freedom are 70 (see above).
4. Ho is rejected if the test statistic is equal to or greater than 1.980.*
5. The t-statistic calculated (see above) is 9.52, so the Ho is *rejected.*
6. Therefore, there *is* a statistical difference between the means of sample 1 and sample 2.

*Obtained from Table 7–8, which presents the distribution of critical values of t. Note the number in the box. The t value will differ, based on the degrees of freedom (based on the sample) and the level of significance required.

by using the tables of t values found in Table 7–8. The researcher will note the degrees of freedom in the left hand column of the table. After locating the degrees of freedom calculated $(N_1 - 1) + (N_2 - 1)$, the researcher will read the number across from that number in the 0.05 (level of significance) column. If the t-test score is larger than the number shown, the null hypothesis will be rejected (meaning that there *is* a significant difference between the two groups of numbers). If the t-test score is smaller than the number shown, the researcher fails to find evidence to reject the null hypothesis meaning that the analysis has not yielded evidence to support rejecting the notion that there is no difference between the means. The null hypothesis is never accepted. One can only fail to reject the null hypothesis.

Simple Analysis of Variance.   The purpose of analysis of variance is similar to the t-test, but it is used to determine if there is a significant difference between the means of *three or more* samples of observations involving interval data. If the analysis provides evidence of a difference between means, an additional test is required to determine exactly which means are different. Use of analysis of variance assumes that the samples are randomly selected (although the ns can be different) and that the variable or variables in question are randomly distributed throughout the population of interest.

Chi Square.   The chi square is a procedure that has a great range of application. It can be used with categories of nominal data that have a relationship but no specific data points. Such relationships may be reported as frequency of occurrence in each category.

The chi square is a method that is used to determine whether the difference between the expected and observed frequencies can be attributed to chance variations in sampling. The test may give distorted results when the expected frequency in any one category is less than five.

Correlation.   While the t-test and analysis of variance determine the differences between and among groups of numbers, correlation designates the degree of relationship or association between two variables or sets of observations using interval data. The correlation coefficient is the index of the relationship between two variables and ranges from −1 to +1, with 0 indicating absolutely no systematic relationship between the variables. For example, when the values in two sets of observations systematically

TABLE 7–8
DISTRIBUTION OF t

df	0.20	0.10	0.05	0.02	0.01	0.001
1	3.078	6.314	12.706	31.821	63.657	636.619
2	1.886	2.920	4.303	6.965	9.925	31.598
3	1.638	2.353	3.182	4.541	5.841	12.941
4	1.533	2.132	2.776	3.747	4.604	8.610
5	1.476	2.015	2.571	3.365	4.032	6.859
6	1.440	1.943	2.447	3.143	3.707	5.959
7	1.415	1.895	2.365	2.998	3.499	5.405
8	1.397	1.860	2.306	2.896	3.355	5.041
9	1.383	1.833	2.262	2.821	3.250	4.781
10	1.372	1.812	2.228	2.764	3.169	4.587
11	1.363	1.796	2.201	2.718	3.106	4.437
12	1.356	1.782	2.179	2.681	3.055	4.318
13	1.350	1.771	2.160	2.650	3.012	4.221
14	1.345	1.761	2.145	2.624	2.977	4.140
15	1.341	1.753	2.131	2.602	2.947	4.073
16	1.337	1.746	2.120	2.583	2.921	4.015
17	1.333	1.740	2.110	2.567	2.898	3.965
18	1.330	1.734	2.101	2.552	2.878	3.922
19	1.328	1.729	2.093	2.539	2.861	3.883
20	1.325	1.725	2.086	2.528	2.815	3.850
21	1.323	1.721	2.080	2.518	2.831	3.819
22	1.321	1.717	2.074	2.508	2.819	3.792
23	1.319	1.714	2.069	2.500	2.807	3.767
24	1.318	1.711	2.064	2.492	2.797	3.745
25	1.316	1.708	2.060	2.485	2.787	3.725
26	1.315	1.706	2.056	2.479	2.779	3.707
27	1.314	1.703	2.052	2.473	2.771	3.690
28	1.313	1.701	2.048	2.467	2.763	3.674
29	1.311	1.699	2.045	2.462	2.756	3.659
30	1.310	1.697	2.042	2.457	2.750	3.646
40	1.303	1.684	2.021	2.423	2.704	3.551
60	1.296	1.671	2.000	2.390	2.660	3.460
120	1.289	1.658	1.980	2.358	2.617	3.373
∞	1.282	1.645	1.960	2.326	2.576	3.291

Table 7–8 is taken from Table III of Fisher & Yates: Statistical Tables for Biological, Agricultural and Medical Research published by Longman Group Ltd. London (previously published by Oliver and Boyd Ltd., Edinburgh) and by permission of the authors and publishers.

increase or decrease *together,* it can be said that there is a *positive* correlation. If the values in one set go up, while the values of the data points in the other one go down, however, a *negative* correlation is said to exist. For example, there is usually a positive correlation between the heights and weights of people. The taller one is, the more likely that person will weigh more, although that is not necessarily true in all cases.

A correlation between two variables does not necessarily mean that one variable causes the other, although with enough such positive correlations over a period of time, causation may be shown. For example, early studies found that the incidence of lung cancer increased with years of heavy smoking. However, not all persons who smoke heavily over many years develop lung cancer, so it could not be said that heavy smoking over many years causes lung cancer. Continued studies over many years, however, have continued to find a positive correlation between heavy smoking and lung cancer, so that smoking is considered a high risk for the development of lung cancer.

While there are numerous types of correlation techniques, only two will be illustrated in this book. These are: (1) rank-order correlation and (2) Pearson-product moment correlation.

Rank-order correlation is easy to determine because it is based on the ranks of a set of numbers. One formula for the calculation of a rank-order method of correlation will be found in Table 7–9. This table demonstrates how to calculate the correlation between temperature reading and radial pulse beat in ten subjects. There should be a positive correlation between these two variables; that is, the higher the temperature, the higher the pulse. A positive correlation of 0.82 (which is very high) was obtained from these ten subjects.

Another popular method for determining correlation is the Pearson-product moment method. One formula for calculating this correlation is presented in Table 7–10. The calculation is somewhat more involved than the rank-order method, but relatively simple if the exact steps are followed as shown in the table. A positive correlation of 0.28 was obtained, which shows a slight correlation between variable X and variable Y.

A specific correlation coefficient may be considered excellent in one situation but not satisfactory in another situation depending on the purpose of the correlation. There are numerous other types of correlation procedures for use with different types of data. The reader is referred to a statistics textbook for this information.

COMPUTER ANALYSIS

All of the statistical formula computations shown in this chapter can easily be performed on a computer in a matter of seconds, even if the sample size is quite large. The beginning researcher is encouraged to utilize university, hospital, or other agency resources for computer analysis if desired. Assistance will be needed from a resource person, nursing researcher colleague, and/or computer staff to learn how to prepare the data for computer analysis. Preparing a computer program, computer time, and/or assistance interpreting the computer analysis will be needed and usually involves a small fee. If the total number of subjects studied is relatively small, however, the sample statistical formulas presented in this chapter can be calculated with a small hand calculator.

TABLE 7–9
RANK-ORDER METHOD OF CORRELATION

$$r = 1 - \frac{6 \Sigma d^2}{N(N^2 - 1)}$$

Subject	(Temperature) Variable X	(Pulse) Variable Y	Rank X	Rank Y	d	d²
1	99	84	5	5	0	0
2	98^4	88	8	4	4	16
3	98^6	80	7	8	1	1
4	100^4	84	4	6	2	4
5	97^8	72	10	9	1	1
6	98^8	82	6	7	1	1
7	100^6	92	3	2	1	1
8	101	96	2	1	1	1
9	98	70	9	10	1	1
10	101^2	90	1	3	2	4
					Σd^2 =	30

$$r = 1 - \frac{6(30)}{10(10^2 - 1)}$$

$$r = 1 - \frac{180}{10(100 - 1)}$$

$$r = 1 - \frac{180}{10(99)}$$

$$r = 1 - \frac{180}{990}$$

$$r = 1 - 0.18$$
$$r = 0.82 \quad \text{(a very high correlation)}$$

SUMMARY

After the collection of the data for a research study, a careful analysis of that data must be made so that generalizations, conclusions, and recommendations can be made by the researcher. The researcher will choose a method of analysis based on the type of data collected *before* the collection of the data.

Measurement is categorized as either *discrete* (*nominal* or *ordinal*) or continuous (*interval* or *ratio*). The statistical procedure selected will depend upon several factors, one of which is the type of measurement possible with the data collected.

Statistical procedures help the researcher to collect, organize, summarize, and analyze quantitative numbers in some way. The two major categories of statistical procedures are *descriptive* and *inferential*.

TABLE 7–10
FORMULA AND SAMPLE OF PEARSON-PRODUCT MOMENT METHOD OF CORRELATION

$$r = \frac{\Sigma xy}{\sqrt{\Sigma x^2 \, \Sigma y^2}}$$

Subject	X variable	Y variable	x	y	x²	y²	xy
1	50	34	4	−8	16	64	−32
2	44	16	−2	−26	4	676	52
3	36	58	−10	16	100	256	−160
4	52	72	6	30	36	900	180
5	18	64	−28	22	784	484	−616
6	15	14	−31	−28	961	784	840
7	31	23	−15	−19	225	361	285
8	62	36	16	−6	256	36	−96
9	70	42	24	0	576	0	0
10	82	61	36	19	1296	361	684

$\Sigma x = 460$ $\Sigma y = 420$ $\Sigma 4^2 = 4254 \Sigma y^2 = 3922$ $\Sigma xy = 1137$
$\bar{x} = 46$ $y = 42$

$$r = \frac{1137}{\sqrt{(4254)\,(3922)}}$$

$$r = \frac{1137}{\sqrt{16684188}}$$

$$r = \frac{1137}{4085}$$

$r = 0.28$ (a slight correlation)

Descriptive techniques help the researcher to describe and organize the data. Some of the simple descriptive procedures that can be used for analyzing data are the: (1) total number, (2) range, and (3) percentages. Measures of central tendency which can be used to describe the data more fully are the: (1) mean, (2) median, (3) mode, (4) standard deviation, and (5) frequency distribution. These types of data can be presented well by using such graphic forms as the: (1) bar graph, (2) histogram, (3) frequency polygon, and (4) pie graph.

Inferential statistics include those statistical procedures that allow the researcher to make specific inferences, generalizations, and/or conclusions from the data. Examples of these procedures are the: (1) t-test, (2) analysis of variance, and (3) chi square, which determine if there are statistically significant differences between and/or among groups of data. The null or statistical hypothesis is used with these procedures. By statistical means, therefore, it is determined if the results could have occurred simply by chance. A 0.05 level of significance (which is usually the minimum acceptable) means that the results could have occurred no more than 5 times out of 100.

Correlation procedures such as the rank-order method of correlation and the Pearson-product movement method of correlation determine the relationship between two variables. A perfect positive correlation is $+1.00$ and a perfect negative correlation is -1.00. A positive correlation means that as one variable increases the other variable increases also. A negative correlation means that as one variable increases, the other variable decreases.

All of the statistical formulas presented in this chapter can be performed by the use of a hand calculator if the number of subjects is relatively small. If large numbers are involved and/or if the beginning researcher desires, these calculations may be performed by a computer in a matter of seconds. Assistance will be needed in preparing the data for the computer and interpreting the final results.

QUESTIONS FOR STUDY AND DISCUSSION

1 Differentiate between discrete and continuous measurement.

2 Give examples of discrete and continuous measurement.

3 What is the difference between descriptive and inferential statistics?

4 Determine the n, $\overline{X}$, Md, and Mo for the following set of numbers.

19	10	25	30	22
16	28	5	20	4
13	20	9	14	17

5 Calculate the S for the above set of numbers.

6 Describe the differences in the histogram, polygon, bar graph, and pie graph.

7 What is the difference between an independent and dependent variable?

8 What is meant by level of significance? What is the normally acceptable minimum level of significance?

9 What does correlation mean?

10 What does a correlation coefficient of 0.80 mean?

REFERENCES

1 John T. Roscoe, *Fundamental Research Statistics,* Holt, Rinehart, and Wilson, New York, 1969, p. 1.

2 Denise F. Polit, and Bernadette P. Hungler, *Nursing Research,* 2d ed., Lippincott, Philadelphia, 1983, p. 483.

3 Frederick J. Kviz, and Kathleen Astin Knafl, *Statistics for Nurses,* Little, Brown, Boston, 1980, p. 138.

BIBLIOGRAPHY

Knapp, Rebecca G., *Basic Statistics for Nurses,* Wiley, New York, 1978.

Kviz, Frederick J., and Knafl, Kathleen Astin, *Statistics for Nurses,* Little, Brown, Boston, 1980.

Roscoe, John T., *Fundamental Research Statistics,* Holt, Rinehart, and Wilson, New York, 1969.

Weiner, Elizabeth Elder, and Daniel L. Weiner, "Understanding the Use of Basic Statistics in Nursing Research," *American Journal of Nursing,* vol. 83, no. 5, 1983, pp. 107–174.

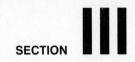

RESEARCH REPORTS

CHAPTER 8

READING AND
EVALUATING
RESEARCH REPORTS

While this book provides a basic introduction for the beginning researcher on how to implement small research studies, another important focus is to provide the nurse with the information needed to find, read, evaluate, and implement research findings in nursing practice. Every professional nurse has the responsibility to be aware of current research findings in order to improve nursing practice. This professional goal will be more and more important in the role of the professional nurse in the future. In fact, the time, effort, and money expended on nursing research will not be well spent if research findings cannot be evaluated and applied in the improvement of patient care. Weiner and Weiner have noted that, "The person who holds the key to making nursing research effective is the nurse who can interpret and use research findings in her daily practice."[1]

Published reports of many research studies, however, are sometimes difficult for the nurse to read and understand clearly because of the basic research and statistical terms used in these reports. It is hoped that the previous chapters on types of research, methodological approaches and designs, and analysis of data will help to clarify and simplify basic research terminology. This chapter will review and utilize much of the terminology presented in previous chapters. The reader is also referred to the glossary in the appendix for review and study of basic research terminology commonly found in research literature.

SELECTING RESOURCES FOR RESEARCH FINDINGS

The most obvious source of completed research studies in nursing is the nursing literature. The major nursing research journals and other published sources of nursing research are discussed in detail in Chapter 4. Most journals have a section for "Letters to

the Editor" or "Incoming Mail." Letters from experienced researchers often are published that give excellent critiques of recently published research. Novice researchers
can learn much about how to evaluate and critique research by routinely reading these
sections.

The nurse is also encouraged to attend seminars, workshops, and symposia where
nurses present their research findings in person. This source provides the nurse with an
opportunity to ask questions directly of the researcher as well as to comment on the
applicability and reasonableness of the conclusions and recommendations for nursing
practice. Some research seminars have a planned oral critique and/or discussion period
immediately following the presentation of each research report. These oral critiques by
experienced nurse researchers will help beginning researchers learn how to evaluate and
discuss research reports in an open and objective manner.

READING A RESEARCH REPORT

Nurses must be able to *read* and *understand* research reports before being able to
evaluate or *critique* them. Leedy[2] has recommended that the reader of research reports
do an overview of the article before reading it in detail. He suggested that the reader: (1)
look at the title, (2) read the abstract, and (3) glance through the report to determine the
various headings and total organization of the report. Then the report can be read in
detail, particularly noting the *problem statement* and *research questions, data collection*
and *interpretation,* and *conclusions.* The nurse who has had minimal experience reading
research reports in the literature should concentrate on the three major areas just listed.
Once these three topics are clearly understood, other details about the report will become
more clear.

In the process of reading, summarizing, and critiquing a research report, it is
suggested that the reader make a personal copy of the article so that the major points can
be underlined or highlighted with a pen or pencil. Comments and questions can also be
written in the margins while reading the report. Most published research reports are not
"light" reading. Research reports may need to be read several times and studied
thoroughly in order to be completely understood. Leedy[2] emphasized that the reader has
"one responsibility: to *know* precisely what the *researcher* has said." The reader cannot
interpret or infer more than what is written by the researcher.

COMPONENTS OF THE REPORT TO BE EVALUATED

Any research report, whether published or presented orally, should be evaluated in detail
to determine the value, importance, and applicability of the results and conclusions and
the implications for nursing practice. The general components of research reports that
should be evaluated are the:

- Title
- Credibility of the researcher
- Abstract
- Problem statement and research questions

- Purpose
- Hypotheses
- Literature review
- Theoretical or conceptual framework
- Research design
- Method of data collection (including informed consent procedures)
- Analysis of data or results (including the use of statistics and graphs)
- Summary and conclusions
- Recommendations and implications for nursing

Title

Many published articles are given titles that will catch the reader's attention. Interesting titles are not necessarily true or effective for research publications, however. The title should clearly, precisely, and completely state the primary focus or essence or key ideas of the research to be discussed. Research article titles tend to be somewhat more lengthy, therefore, because of the need to include the major components of the research study being reported. Veldman noted that, "A good title should identify the major *variables* (not their operational definitions) and the *populations* (not the specific samples) to be studied."[3]

Titles often emerge or are changed after the manuscript has been completed. Although the title does not affect the value of the study itself, the title may not clearly describe the essence of the study. This problem is more one of writing and editing than research. However, if the title is not clear, it may be that the problem is not clearly defined or the study completely described.

Credibility of the Researcher

The reader of written research publications should routinely review the credentials of the author/researcher. Usually a brief description of the author is included with the article. This description may include degrees, experience, and current position. Questions that can be asked to aid in evaluating the credibility of the researcher are:

- Is the researcher a nurse?
- What is the researcher's specific educational preparation?
  In research?
  In the content area being studied?
- What kinds of professional experiences has the researcher had?
  In research?
  In clinical practice?
- Has the researcher conducted and/or published other reports of research studies? If so, how effective have they been?
- Does the researcher present a clear, concise, systematic, and organized report?

Although doctoral and postdoctoral preparation are assumed to be the educational levels with a major focus on research, one must not assume that doctoral preparation assures valid studies. Because historically the doctoral preparation of nurses has varied considerably in terms of schools and fields of study, the amount and types of research preparation in these programs vary greatly. Many nurses who have completed a recent master's degree in nursing with a strong clinical *and* research focus, for example, may generate excellent ideas for research and conduct well-planned and valid studies.

Abstract

The abstract should contain a clear and succinct overview of the study in about 100 to 150 words. The purpose, methodological approach used, brief description of subjects, conclusions, and implications should be included. Not all published research articles will contain an abstract, but most of the articles in research journals will have an abstract at the beginning of the study.

Problem Statement and Research Questions

The problem statement and research question(s) are the most important components of the evaluation because if these are not clear, the remaining sections of the research, and the report, are likely to be fuzzy and weak. The reviewer of research articles should have the following questions in mind while reading and evaluating the problem statement. Is the problem:

- Clear, concrete, and concisely stated?
- Easily communicated to others?
- Researchable?
- Related to observable events?
- Significant to nursing?
- Important enough to be studied?

Other questions about the study related to the problem statement are listed below.

- What need is being met by this study?
- Was it worth the financial expenditures used?
- Are the results and conclusions worth the time and effort spent on the study?
- Are the results generalizable to other situations and/or areas?

The problem statement and research questions must be so specific and clear that anyone who has no knowledge of the field of study would be able to understand them. The problem statement presents the overall focus of the study. The research questions evolve from the problem statement and are much more specific.

Purpose

A specific purpose may or may not be stated. If it is stated, it expands on the problem statement. The purpose presents "the reasons why the problem is worth studying—the justification for the expenditure of resources."[4] The ultimate purpose of clinical nursing research, for example, is to improve patient and client care. The purpose of any *clinical* nursing study, therefore, should be related in some way to the improvement of nursing care.

Hypotheses

If the study design is one of an experimental or quasi-experimental type, research or null (statistical) hypotheses will be stated. There may be one or more major hypotheses with several subhypotheses for each major hypothesis. Descriptive studies may or may not have stated hypotheses. If the study has involved the collection of quantitative data of some type, hypotheses will be tested statistically if the sample of subjects is large enough. If, however, the design is qualitative in type, or if only percentages are used for summarization of data in a quantitative descriptive study, hypotheses cannot be used because they cannot be tested. The reader is referred to Chapter 7 for a review of the testing of hypotheses.

Hypotheses should be stated clearly and include all elements of what is being tested in the most succinct way possible. Hypotheses may be stated in a research or null (statistical) form, although the research form is preferred because it is less awkward and confusing than the null form. Most important, of course, is the fact that the hypotheses must be directly derived from the research questions.

Literature Review

Several major questions need to be asked about the literature review. Most of these questions are derived from the detailed discussion of the literature in Chapter 4. For example:

- Is the review organized and comprehensive?
- Have the references been published within the last three to five years?
- Does the discussion proceed from the general to the specific?
- Do the references relate specifically to the problem statement?
- Are classic studies related to the topic included?
- Are positive and negative findings discussed objectively?
- Are the references documented consistently?

The literature review does not need to be lengthy, but it should flow well and provide the reader with a clear understanding about the background of the problem being studied. Most of all, the review should *not* simply be a collection of disconnected summaries of remotely related studies. The studies need to be related to the problem being studied, flow from one idea to the next, and present a central theme.[5]

Theoretical or Conceptual Framework

The discussion of the theoretical or conceptual framework upon which the study is based may be included as a part of the section on the literature review or it may be a separate section. In either case, the reader will look for a concise, clear discussion of the theory or major concepts that include a brief historical perspective and rationale for use of the theory or concepts with the particular study being reported. The following questions can be asked about the framework:

- Does the theoretical or conceptual framework lend structural support to the research?

- Is the theoretical or conceptual framework appropriate for the problem (question)?
- Is the theoretical or conceptual framework understandable?
- Is the overall framework presented as well as its associated theoretical components?

Research Design

The specific design should be clearly identified; for example experimental, quasi-experimental, descriptive, historical. If there are adaptations in design, these should be discussed. The design should be appropriate for the research questions. For example, if the research question involves evaluating the effectiveness of a new nursing approach not normally in use, the new approach will need to be compared with the nursing approach in current use so an experimental or quasi-experimental design would be appropriate.

Method of Data Collection

The method of data collection must fit the design. For example, if an experimental design is selected, the random selection of subjects must be utilized, considering the design, method of collecting data, and method of analyzing the data.

The complete methodology should be discussed in detail, from pilot study to specific method of analyzing the data. If specific instruments were selected or developed for the collection of data, a discussion of the validity and reliability of the instruments used should be included. Downs and Newman[6] noted that, "Justification must be based on firm evidence beyond arguments that the tool is 'the best available' or 'has been used frequently.' " If validity or reliability of the tools are not discussed in the report, it probably means that they have not been determined.

There should be a complete discussion of the selection of subjects (number, description, criteria for selection, and method of selection) as well as informed consent procedures used. Extraneous variables that might have affected the results should be identified and discussed.

Specific questions that can be asked about the methodology are:

- Is the method of data collection clearly identified?
- Is the method of data collection consistent with the identified problem?
- Is the method of data collection appropriate for the chosen conceptual or theoretical framework?

Analysis of Data or Results

The type of data obtained (qualitative or quantitative) should be discussed. The statistical procedures used to analyze the data will be identified and described. Results of statistical procedures should be presented in as clear a method as possible. The reader is referred to Chapter 7 for a discussion of major statistical procedures, standard abbreviations and formulas used in the procedures, and concepts such as levels of statistical significance.

It is not expected that the beginning researcher will be able to determine whether or not the correct statistical procedure was used without advanced study and experience in statistics. A colleague, experienced researcher, or consultant can be utilized to assist with this type of evaluation if needed or desired.

The use of tables, figures, and/or graphs (bar, histogram, polygon, and pie) empha- size the major statistical results. These tables, figures, and graphs must be labeled clearly (title, horizontal, and vertical axis) and discussed in the text. Careful readers often find errors or inconsistencies in tables or graphs, even though the specific statistical pro- cedures utilized are not clearly understood.

The following questions can be asked about the analysis of the data:

- Are procedures used for analyzing the data presented in detail?
- Is sufficient data presented to validate the researcher's conclusions?
- Does the data relate to the generation of a theory?
- If the research utilizes a qualitative approach, does the data support the evidence through the use of vivid descriptions such as:
  Sights and sounds
  Direct quotations
  Dramatic segments of the field notes
  Personal case studies
  Background descriptions

Most important of all, it must be determined if the data support or do not support the hypotheses.

Summary and Conclusions

The summary should clearly and concisely discuss the problem statement, hypotheses, theoretical/conceptual framework, design, methodology, analysis of data, and findings. Sometimes this section is called the *discussion*. The conclusion discusses the *major* findings, particularly those which answer the research questions and determine accep- tance or rejection of the previously stated hypotheses. "So what?" is a typical question the reviewer should ask when evaluating the conclusions. The most important evaluation of the conclusions is to determine whether or not *the conclusions are based on the findings*. The conclusions must be objective and not be influenced by the researcher's preferences, experiences, or ideas.

The researcher may also discuss omissions or weaknesses in the study at this point. The researcher's identification and sharing of these weaknesses adds to the value of the report because the reader is given more information to use in determining the applicabil- ity of the findings.[7]

Recommendations and Implications for Nursing

Finally, the last section will include any recommendations the researcher wants to make, including the implications for nursing. The recommendations may include suggestions for nursing (if the findings confirm them) and/or recommendations about the research study itself such as: (1) repeating the study with a larger number or different type of selection of subjects, (2) repeating the study with specific variables controlled, and/or (3) repeating the study in a different geographic location.

The conclusions should lead to a statement about the implications of the findings for nursing. If the research is *nursing research,* there should be identifiable implications for some area of nursing. The implications should be stated clearly and discussion about the generalizability of the findings included. Sometimes a researcher "is tempted to generalize beyond the population on which the study is based."[8] For this reason, the reader especially needs to understand thoroughly the problem and method of subject selection. At this point, the reader may need to refer to the discussion of these topics in the report.

Finally, beginning researchers and/or practicing nurses must determine, based on the detailed evaluation guidelines just presented, whether the findings, recommendations, and nursing implications are valid and important enough to incorporate the research results into their nursing practice. This evaluative process will be discussed in Chapter 10. A sample tool which can be used to evaluate the major components of a *quantitative* research report may be found in Table 8-1. Criteria for the assessment of a *qualitative* research study may be found in Table 8–2.

SUMMARY

All professional nurses have a responsibility to read, review, and evaluate the literature in nursing research even though they do not conduct studies themselves. Sources of nursing research are the nursing journals, books reporting nursing research, and seminars, workshops, and symposia where nurse researchers present their findings in person.

While reading research studies or listening to oral research reports, the beginning researcher and practicing nurse should look for and critically evaluate the following components of the research process: (1) title, (2) credibility of the researcher, (3) problem statement and research questions, (4) purpose, (5) hypotheses, (6) literature review, (7) theoretical or conceptual framework, (8) research design, (9) method of collecting data and informed consent procedures, (10) analysis of data including the use of statistics and graphs, (11) summary and conclusions, and (12) recommendations and implications for nursing.

After studying the above components in a published or oral research study, nurses can decide whether or not to utilize the findings and implement the recommendations in their nursing careers. A sample tool was presented which will give the nurse guidelines to help in this evaluation process.

QUESTIONS FOR STUDY AND DISCUSSION

1 Where can the practicing nurse find recent studies in nursing research?

2 Is the title of a research study important? Why or why not?

3 What factors should be considered in evaluating the credibility of the nurse researcher/author?

4 Which of the twelve components of a research study discussed in this chapter could be considered the most important?

5 Is the research hypothesis or the null hypothesis used most often in published research studies? Why?

TABLE 8–1
SAMPLE TOOL TO EVALUATE THE MAJOR COMPONENTS OF A QUANTITATIVE
RESEARCH STUDY

Points	Components	Criteria	Evaluation
3	Title	Is the title: . . . clear? . . . precise? . . . reflective of the problem of the study?	Yes__ (1) No__ Yes__ (1) No__ Yes__ (1) No__
4	Researcher	Is the researcher qualified in subject area by: . . . education? . . . experience?	Yes__ (2) No__ Yes__ (2) No__
15	Problem statement/ research questions	Is the problem statement/research question(s): . . . clear, complete, and concisely stated?* . . . significant to nursing? . . . operationally defined?	Yes__ (5) No__ Yes__ (5) No__ Yes__ (5) No__
10	Purpose	Is the purpose clearly stated?	Yes__ (2) No__
	Hypotheses (If no hypotheses, count purpose as 10 points)	Are the hypotheses: . . . appropriate for the problem statement? . . . appropriate for the design? . . . clear and concisely stated? . . . testable by quantifiable data? . . . capable of answering the research questions?	 Yes__ (3) No__ Yes__ (2) No__ Yes__ (1) No__ Yes__ (1) No__ Yes__ (1) No__
6	Theoretical/ conceptual framework (If no theoretical/ conceptual frame-work identified, add 6 points to literature review as indicated with a +)	Does it provide a clear framework for the study? Is there a rationale for the use of the particular framework?	Yes__ (3) No__ Yes__ (3) No__
7	Literature Review	Do the references relate to the problem statement? Is the review comprehensive? Does the review use only primary sources? Have the references been published within the past three to five years? Are the references documented com-pletely and consistently?	Yes__ (2) No__ +(2) Yes__ (2) No__ +(1) Yes__ (1) No__ +(1) Yes__ (1) No__ +(1) Yes__ (1) No__ +(1)

TABLE 8–1 (continued)
SAMPLE TOOL TO EVALUATE THE MAJOR COMPONENTS OF A QUANTITATIVE RESEARCH STUDY

Points	Components	Criteria	Evaluation
10	Design	Is the design identified by name and described?	Yes__ (5) No__
		Is the design appropriate for the research questions?	Yes__ (5) No__
20	Methodology	Does the methodology fit the design?	Yes__ (2) No__
		Is the methodology discussed in detail?	Yes__ (2) No__
		Is the method of data collection appropriate to the problem?	Yes__ (2) No__
		Are the instruments used	
		. . . valid?	Yes__ (2) No__
		. . . reliable?	Yes__ (2) No__
		Is the method of selecting subjects clear?	Yes__ (2) No__
		Were there an adequate number of subjects in the study?	Yes__ (2) No__
		Were informed consent procedures used?	Yes__ (2) No__
		Were the major variables:	
		. . . identified?	Yes__ (2) No__
		. . . controlled?	Yes__ (2) No__
8	Analysis of Data	Are the statistical procedures used to analyze the data clearly identified?	Yes__ (2) No__
		Are tables, figures, and/or graphs:	
		. . . used?	Yes__ (2) No__
		. . . clearly labeled?	Yes__ (2) No__
		. . . discussed?	Yes__ (2) No__
10	Summary and conclusions	Is the summary clear and concise?	Yes__ (5) No__
		Are the conclusions clear and based on the findings?*	Yes__ (5) No__
7	Recommendations and implications for nursing	Are generalizations appropriate to the research design and sampling techniques used?*	Yes__ (5) No__
		Are the stated implications for nursing clear and reasonable?	Yes__ (1) No__
		Are recommendations made to replicate and/or revise the study?	Yes__ (1) No__

HOW THE TOOL CAN BE USED TO EVALUATE A RESEARCH STUDY:

1. Yes—Positive Components
   No—Negative Components

2. Add up the Yes points in parentheses ____

3. Estimated evaluations based on number of *Yes* answers
   90–100 Excellent
   80–90 Good
   70–80 Fair
   ↓ 70 Questionable

*4. Essential *Yes* Components
   If these items are not checked yes, the research report is questionable.

TABLE 8–2
ASSESSMENT CRITERIA FOR EVALUATING INDUCTIVE RESEARCH STUDIES FOR THE GENERATION OF QUALITATIVE DATA*

1. The Researcher

   What is the credibility and the credentials of the researcher?
   Does the researcher demonstrate a confidence in the credibility of the research?
   Does the researcher present a clear, concise, systematic ordering of the data analysis?

2. General Overall Concerns

   Is the purpose of the research presented in a clear concise manner in conjunction with the social or empirical world in which the research is to take place?
   Does the researcher offer a logical and clear picture of the research proposed by offering a guiding perspective?
   Does the researcher demonstrate a research direction by either specifically stating a problem (question) or moving toward a problem area?
   Does the research suggest some degree of hypothesizing although an hypothesis is not succinctly identified?

3. Theoretical or Conceptual Framework (Not a requirement)

   Does the theoretical or conceptual framework lend support to the proposed research?
   Is the theoretical or conceptual framework appropriate for the problem being proposed?
   Is the theoretical or conceptual framework understandable (in social science terminology)?
   Is the overall framework as well as its associated theoretical statements presented?

4. Data

   Is the method of collecting the data clearly identified?
   Is the method of collecting data consistent with the problem of the research or the problem area that is identified?
   Is the method of collecting the data appropriate for the chosen conceptual framework?
   Does the researcher describe the data of the social world in a vivid manner?
   If the purpose of the research is to generate theory of a substantive nature, does the description of the data relate to the generation of a theory?
   Is sufficient data presented to validate the researcher's conclusions?
   Does the data support the evidence through the use of vivid descriptions, that is, the use of sight and sounds such as:

   A. Direct quotations
   B. Dramatic segments of the field notes
   C. Personal case studies
   D. Background descriptions

   Is a codified procedure for analyzing the data presented, that is, use of the constant comparative method or standard analytical procedures?

5. Developing a Theory

   Does the presented theory fit the substantive area in which it will be used?
   Is the theory understandable to lay persons concerned with the area?
   Is the theory sufficiently general to be applicable to a multitude of diverse daily situations within the substantive area?
   Does the theory provide the potential user the partial control over the structure and process of daily situations as they change through time?

TABLE 8–2 (continued)
ASSESSMENT CRITERIA FOR EVALUATING INDUCTIVE RESEARCH STUDIES FOR THE
GENERATION OF QUALITATIVE DATA*

6. Judging Credibility of the Research from the Reader's Perspective

Does the reader feel that he/she vicariously was also in the field?
Does the reader feel that his/her assessments are similar to those of the researcher's and the
    conclusions were similarly derived?
Is the reader able to follow the researcher's codified procedure for analyzing the data?
Is the theory able to be qualified by the reader?

    A. Is the theory correct?
    B. Can the theory be adjusted to fit the diverse conditions of different social structures?
    C. Can the theory be invalidated through the reader's experience or knowledge?
    D. Is the theory deemed inapplicable to other kinds of structures?

*Criteria used for judging, or evaluating quantitative research cannot be used for evaluating the merits of qualitative,
inductive research studies.

    6 What are four major questions which should be asked about the literature review?
    7 What are three components of the research methodology which should be evaluated?
    8 What is the most important factor to evaluate in the summary and conclusions section of a research report?
    9 What types of recommendations are usually made in research studies?
    10 Who decides whether the implications for nursing discussed at the end of a research study are important and realistic?

REFERENCES

1 Elizabeth Elder Weiner, and Daniel L. Weiner, "Understanding the Use of Basic Statistics in Nursing Research," *American Journal of Nursing,* vol. 83, no. 5, 1983, p. 770.
2 Paul D. Leedy, *How to Read Research and Understand It,* Macmillan, New York, 1981, pp. 29–32.
3 Donald J. Veldman, *Writing a Thesis or Dissertation Proposal in the Behavioral Sciences,* American Continental, Fort Worth, Texas, 1971, p. 1.
4 Veldman, ibid., p. 7.
5 Veldman, ibid., p. 9.
6 Florence S. Downs, and Margaret A. Newman, *A Source of Nursing Research,* 2d ed., Davis, Philadelphia, 1978, p. 8.
7 Downs and Newman, ibid., p. 12.
8 Downs and Newman, ibid., p. 11.

BIBLIOGRAPHY

Downs, Florence S., *A Source Book of Nursing Research,* 3d ed., Davis, Philadelphia, 1984.
Fleming, Juanita W., and Hayter, Jean, "Reading Research Reports Critically," *Nursing Outlook,* vol. 22, no. 3, 1974, pp. 172–175.
Polit, Denise F., and Hungler, Bernadette, P.: *Nursing Research,* Lippincott, Philadelphia, 1983, pp. 581–593.

CHAPTER 9

PRESENTING AND WRITING RESEARCH-RELATED REPORTS

The ability to communicate well, both orally and in writing, is an essential requirement for any person who wants to function effectively and advance in his or her profession. As nurses become more involved in assessing patient and client needs, studying health care problems, and proposing plans to meet those needs and problems, both in the inpatient and outpatient care settings, they will need to be precise and articulate in their communication skills. Because nurses are in unique positions to be aware of problems and needs in the health care delivery system, they can perform assessments, surveys, scientific observations, and specific research studies on these problems and needs in efforts to change health care policy.

Extensive data about problems may be collected and analyzed by the nurse. Excellent recommendations proposed for change may be realistic and supported by the data. However, unless the results and recommendations are communicated effectively to the individuals or groups who have the ability, power, and/or financial resources to make the suggested changes, nurses' recommendations will not be well received. It is important, therefore, that nurses learn to prepare oral and written reports of problem-solving and research findings that will communicate in a clear, concise, and appropriate manner the results and recommendations of their studies.

ORGANIZING THE REPORT

Whether the report is to be a written or oral one, some of the same ideas apply. The report should flow in a logical and organized manner. If the report is of a completed research study, for example, the content will start with a strong introduction that leads to the problem and ends with the conclusions and recommendations. One phase will logically flow to the next to provide a total overview of the report.

An initial topical outline will be very helpful. The outline can be very broad or quite detailed. Either way, the outline helps the writer to organize his or her thoughts and the major points to be made. After a draft of the report has been written, the writer can refer to the outline to determine if all the major ideas have been included. An outline often saves time eventually because it keeps the writer from having to reorganize and rewrite a report that does not seem to flow well. An outline is even more important for an oral report because it breaks up the report into several phases, making it easier for the presenter to speak and for the listeners to follow.

The nurse also should take into consideration to whom the report is to be given. For example, if a completed research report is to be presented orally to a university-wide group of faculty and students from disciplines other than nursing, the report should clearly state the problem and the conclusions in lay terminology that will be understood by persons other than nurses. The methodology will more likely be understood by nonnursing faculty and students; and in fact they may have more questions about methodology than about the problem and the content of the study. If, on the other hand, the nurse is presenting a completed research study to nursing faculty, nursing students and/or health agency staff, nursing terminology will be used as well as the specific methodology of the study.

THE WRITTEN REPORT

Types of research-related reports that students may need to write are:

- Summaries of published research studies
- Critiques or evaluations of published research studies
- Statements of problems and/or research questions identified in clinical areas which need to be studied
- Reviews of literature related to the problems to be studied
- Research proposals
- Completed research projects

Practicing nurses may want or need to write one or more of the following:

- Proposals for change based on the collection and analysis of data on a problem encountered in the clinical area
- Research proposals of a study the nurse wants to conduct in the clinical unit
- Grant proposals
- Completed research projects with recommendations based on their study findings
- Research abstracts

The Research Proposal

A research proposal is a written plan that gives essential details about why and how the study is to be conducted. Research proposals vary in format and length, depending upon the setting. In general, the proposal should be clear and complete so that anyone reading it will be able to understand what is intended even if they are not familiar with the problem to be studied. There is often a temptation, after identification of a problem that

TABLE 9.1
TYPICAL OUTLINE FOR A RESEARCH PROPOSAL

Title Page

Table of Contents

Introduction

Purpose of the Study

Statement of the Problem

The Research Questions

Definition of Terms

Hypotheses

Review of the Literature or Background of the Study

Theoretical or Conceptual Framework

Research Design

Methodology or Procedures for Data Collection

Analysis of the Data or Procedures for Data Analysis

References

Bibliography

Appendices

---

needs study, to start collecting data about the problem. However, if the problem is not completely clear, or if the problem has already been studied by others, time will be wasted if data are collected too soon because the wrong data may be collected from the wrong populations. The research proposal forces the researcher to clarify the problem, to determine what studies have been completed previously on the same topic, and to make explicit methodological plans to study the problem. A typical outline for a relatively simple research proposal is presented in Table 9-1.

The introduction should be relatively brief and lead to the statement of the problem. The purpose, problem statement, research question, and hypothesis are discussed in detail in Chapter 3. The literature review is discussed in Chapter 4. Only classic samples of the related literature should be included in the research proposal rather than all of the literature reviewed. The theoretical or conceptual framework for the study will probably evolve out of the literature review. Research design and methodology are discussed in Chapters 5 and 6. These last two topics should be discussed thoroughly in the research proposal.

The proposed methods of analyzing the data (see Chapter 7) should be explained and very clearly written in the proposal. Data collected may not be usable unless it is clear how the data are to be analyzed before they are collected. The references or footnotes (those sources quoted or paraphrased) and the bibliography (other general related references) should also be included in the proposal.

The total proposal is written in the *future tense* and should be complete and approved by those who need to approve it (for example, instructors, research committees, or clinical agencies) before any portion of it is implemented. The process of having a proposal approved is discussed in detail in Chapter 10.

Grant Proposals

Almost any kind of research will require the expenditure of some amount of money. Expenses are incurred for typing, duplicating, travel, computer services, possibly equipment, and perhaps consultation. Students who are enrolled in research or honors courses may be required to initiate and complete an independent research project that will require supplies and/or equipment. Practicing nurses employed by agencies may be able to order essential research supplies and equipment through their own department for small problem-solving studies, but if the project is more extensive, specific outside funding may be needed. Sources of funding are discussed in Chapter 11. The purpose of this section is to present suggestions for preparing and writing the formal request for research funds.

As with the research proposal, it is important to find out who is going to review the request for funds and act on it. If the request for funds is being presented to peers, such as a nursing research committee, for example, nursing terminology (but not professional jargon or abbreviations) should be used. If, on the other hand, the request is being submitted to a local volunteer community organization (such as the Women's League) or a private foundation, the request should not include terms used only in nursing. This does not mean that the proposal should be written in terms that any person can understand, but that it be written in language that the educated layman can easily understand. The writer should not insult or try to impress the reviewers, but should write clearly and objectively.

Regardless of who is to review the proposal, the request should be clearly written and follow the guidelines provided (if any) exactly. For this reason, the researcher should write an exploratory letter to the funding agency to determine if they fund studies on the topic being proposed and to request a copy of their guidelines. If possible, a telephone call or personal visit with one of the persons who represents the funding agency is also helpful. Sometimes there are representatives of the organization or agency in the local community so that travel is not necessary.

Guidelines for requesting research funds differ greatly. The guidelines may request a copy of the complete research proposal in addition to a specific budget and monthly plan of activities, or they may require only a two or three page description of the proposed study. A typical outline for a grant proposal will be found in Table 9–2. The most important parts of the written request for funding are the:

- Overall goals and objectives
  Is the purpose of the study very clear and stated in a manner that can be easily understood by someone not familiar with the content?
  Are the goals and objectives specific?
  Are the goals and objectives realistic and obtainable?
  Are the goals and objectives congruent with the funding agency's goals and objectives?
- Expected outcomes
  What is expected to have happened at the end of the study?
  Are the expected outcomes congruent with the goals and objectives?
  Are the expected outcomes proposed worthwhile?
- Budget
  How much total money is requested for one year?

TABLE 9.2
TYPICAL OUTLINE FOR APPLICATIONS FOR RESEARCH FUNDING

1. Cover Sheet
2. Abstract (short overview of study)
3. Table of Contents
4. Narrative Description
    Introduction
    Statement of the Problem and Research Questions
    Overall Goals and Objectives
    Literature Review
    Procedures/Methodology/Proposed Solution/Implementation
    Expected Outcomes
    Rationale or Significance
    Methods of Dissemination of Results
    Organization and Management Plan Including a Graphic Schedule
    Staff
    Facilities
    Method of Evaluation
5. Proposed Budget
    Personnel
    Consultants
    Supplies and Expenses
    Equipment
    Travel
    Space
6. Appendix
Resumes/Vitae (Short)
References and Bibliography (Brief)
Letters of endorsement or support (Optional)

Is the amount reasonable based on the expected outcomes?
Is it clear exactly how every dollar is to be used?
Who will be responsible for receiving, controlling, and expending the funds?
Is the requested budget sufficient to meet the goals and objectives?

The request for funds should be adequate to complete the project as planned considering inflation (for example, the increase in cost of travel or postage) and unexpected emergencies. One should not ask for much more than needed, however, with the belief that what is actually needed will then be received (good reviewers notice excessive requests). Nor should one ask for too little, which could show that the project is not worth more money or that the stated goals and objectives cannot be met with the amount of funds requested.

Other components of the written proposal for funding usually include the following:

• A statement of the problem and/or research questions to be answered that will clarify the overall goals and objectives.

• A literature review that should not be lengthy, but that should include essential references that support the need for the study.

• A discussion of the procedures and methodology that should be relatively short and very clear.

• The process of evaluation that should be related to the goals and objectives.

• Methods of dissemination of the results to others for application.

• An organization and management plan, including a description of facilities available to help carry out the project and a graphic schedule of the major tasks from the beginning to the end of the funding period (a sample of a graphic or time schedule is shown in Figure 9–1).

In addition, some information can be included in the appendix that may or may not specifically be requested in the guidelines. The information will be available if needed, but it will not add to the length of the main proposal itself. Reviewers usually have multiple proposals to study and they do not have time to review long written proposals that include more information than that listed in the guidelines. The appendix should be well labeled and on colored paper so that it can easily be differentiated from the main body of the proposal. Examples of content for the appendix are:

FIGURE 9–1
Sample graphic or time schedule.

Months

Month	Jan.	Feb.	March	April	May	June	July	August	Sept.	Oct.	Nov.	Dec.
Analyze and summarize pilot study data	▨	▨										
Revise instrument based on pilot study statistics			▨									
Identify and locate possible subjects			▨	▨	▨	▨	▨	▨				
Collect data (subject interviews)				▨	▨	▨	▨	▨	▨			
Analyze and summarize final data										▨	▨	
Prepare final report and manuscripts for publication												▨

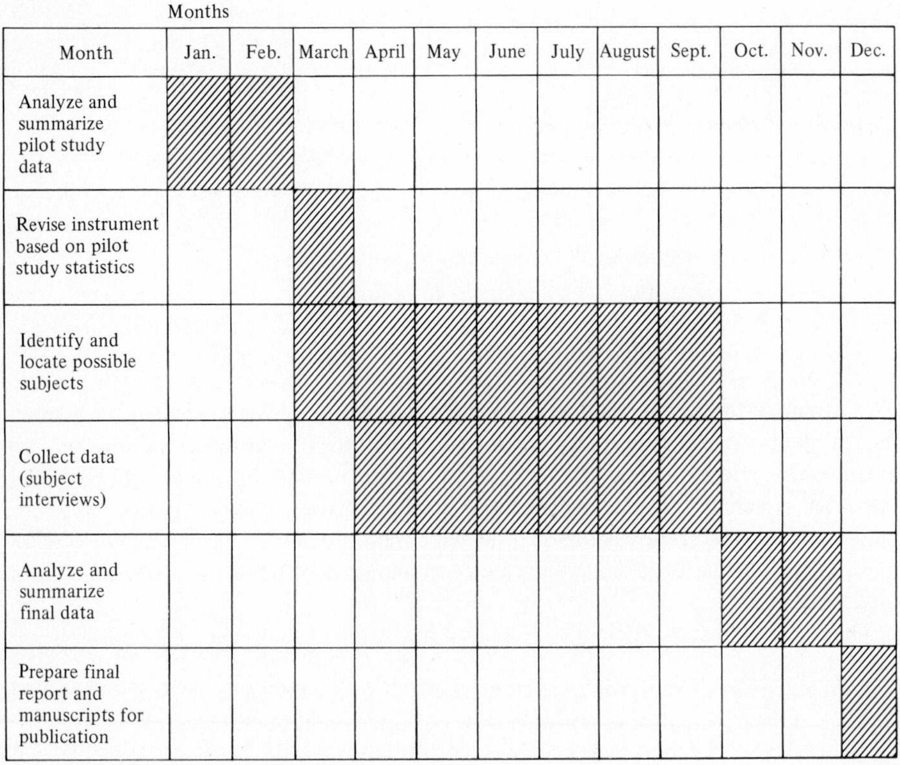

- Resumes/vitae of the person or persons who will be conducting the study.
- Bibliography of related literature only if absolutely needed. It should not be made lengthy in an attempt to impress the reviewers.
- Letters of endorsement, support, and/or approvals from teachers, supervisors, safeguards in human research committees, and clinical agencies to be utilized for the research.
- Maps of geographical areas such as census tracts.
- Floor plans of hospital units, if applicable.

After the proposal for funding has been prepared, it is helpful to check it against the guidelines again and to proofread it for any possible spelling or typing errors. As with all written reports, the more professional appearing the proposal, the more likely it is to be given serious consideration for funding. The required number of copies should be made and the application should be delivered or mailed so that it *arrives* at the funding agency *before* the deadline. Most agencies will not consider requests which arrive after the deadline.[1]

The Research Report

The research report, which is different from the research proposal, is a systematic written report of the completed research study. Much of the content of the research proposal will be utilized in the final report. However, the report is written in the *past tense* because the study will have been completed. A sample outline for a completed research project will be found in Table 9–3. Not all of the topics listed in Table 9–3 will be needed for every research report, depending upon the methodological approach used. For example, the definition of terms may be unnecessary and there may be no stated hypotheses.

The literature review will be more extensive in the final report than in the research proposal. The relationship of the theoretical or conceptual framework to the problem being studied will be discussed. The research design and methodology will be presented in detail. Analysis of the data will include the specific data collected and the results of the statistical analysis. The use of tables, figures, and graphs (see Chapter 7) will enhance this area of the report. The discussion of the findings will describe what the statistical results mean in descriptive terms. Other pertinent findings will also be discussed. The conclusion includes the major summary of the findings and attempts to answer the question "So what?" The recommendations discuss if and how the conclusions will affect nursing practice as well as identify areas for further study, if appropriate. For example, perhaps the researcher will recommend that the study be repeated with a different size sample or that the methodology be revised so that a specific variable will be controlled.

Research Abstracts

An abstract in general is a brief (usually 100 to 500 words) summary of a study, manuscript, journal article, or book that includes the major points of the work. Research abstracts briefly summarize the essential elements of a study. Fuller[2] has described the research abstract as a concise (150–200 words) summary that "has three major parts: a

TABLE 9.3
SAMPLE OUTLINE FOR A COMPLETED RESEARCH REPORT

Title Page

Table of Contents

List of Tables

List of Figures

Introduction

Purpose of the Study

Statement of the Problem

The Research Questions

Definition of Terms

Hypotheses

Review of the Literature

Theoretical or Conceptual Framework

Research Design

Methodology

Analysis of the Data

Discussion of Findings

Conclusions

Recommendations

References

Bibliography

Appendices

statement of the problem, a short description of design and methods, and a summary and interpretation of the results of the study." The research abstract at the beginning of an article helps readers to determine if they want to read the complete report. Research abstracts are also used to help planners evaluate prospective research reports for possible presentations at meetings and seminars. Sources of published research abstracts are discussed in Chapter 4.

The researcher, therefore, will usually need to prepare an abstract to accompany the longer written research report. Because the abstract is written after the long report, it would seem fairly easy to write a brief summary. However, condensing many months of work and perhaps hundreds of pages into 200 words or less can be a challenge. Samples of two different types of abstracts may be found in Appendix F (Short Form) and Appendix G (Long Form).

Helpful Writing Hints

Whether the written report is a brief summary of a published research study (see Chapter 8) on a 5 × 8 card or a report of a completed research project, there are several very practical suggestions that will improve the final written report.

Follow Guidelines.   If there are specific guidelines required by the instructor (for a course), or requested by a hospital research committee (for approval), or provided by a funding agency (for a grant), the nurse should *follow those guidelines explicitly,* even to the outline format (for example, 1, 2, 3, 4; a, b, c, d) and typing instructions (for example, 1-in. margins). Usually there are specific criteria used to evaluate papers or proposals that are based on the guidelines. If the guidelines are not followed exactly, the persons who review the paper or proposal will have difficulty evaluating it and, therefore, acceptance may be less likely.

Writing Style.   A clear, concise, and readable writing style is essential in any report. Many beginning writers make an error trying to write in a "scholarly" manner, especially when writing a research-related report. Scholarly does *not* mean using many long words with obscure meanings, however. Florence Downs, the editor of *Nursing Research,* emphasized this point in an editorial: ". . . authors seem to misunderstand . . . that a published work is judged to be scholarly by virtue of its content, not its verbiage."[3]

A few suggestions to consider when writing reports are presented in Table 9–4. A good unabridged dictionary; a dictionary of foreign terms; a handbook of synonyms, antonyms, and prepositions; an encyclopedia; and a thesaurus are excellent resources to have readily available when writing formal reports and manuscripts. References that can be used to improve writing skills are included in the chapter bibliography.

Tables, Graphs, and Figures.   The use of tables, graphs, and figures adds much to a final report, especially if there are numerical data that can be illustrated in this way. A table or a graph will demonstrate a major finding in a much more clear manner than will a long narrative with a detailed description of numbers. The major point of the table or graph should be discussed briefly in the narrative description, however. If two or more numbers are being compared, they should be placed in a table or graph.

A table or a figure can be used for comparing numbers, listing ideas, or describing sets of events. Graphs are more commonly used for displaying numerical data. The most common types of graphs used are the: (1) bar graph, (2) histogram, (3) pie graph, and (4) frequency polygon. These are described and illustrated in Chapter 7.

However, an incomplete table or graph is useless. A clear and complete graph will include:

- An identifying number
- A complete descriptive title
- An accurately labeled vertical axis
- An accurately labeled horizontal axis
- Numerical intervals appropriate to the range
- References (for example, where the data was obtained)
- Appropriate use of vertical and horizontal lines based on the writing manual used

Bibliography Format.   A *complete* and *consistent* bibliographical format should be used in any formal paper. There are many styles to use. If the university, hospital, publisher, or other agency requires a specific format, that is what should be used. In most

TABLE 9.4
WRITING SUGGESTIONS

Positive Points	Negative Components
Write clearly what you want to say.	Use of flowery, fancy, or archaic words (such as heretofor, aforementioned)
Write for your reader (experienced researcher or nursing students).	
Use active words.	Use of passive voice (a decision is made by researchers)
Check all questionable spelling (commitment, judgment, memento, mucus, mucous)	Use of sexist language (The nurse . . . she)
	Use of professional jargon (such as Bardex, output)
Use punctuation correctly (better to underuse than overuse).	
	Use of meaningless words (such as actual)
	Use of unnecessary words (It is related to the fact that . . .)
Use words correctly (such as a medical *regimen* and a political *regime*).	Use of words that imply prejudice (such as "senile" old man)
	Use of cliches (such as "good as gold")
	Use of the real names of patients or simulated ethnic names
	Including specific dates, names of institutions, or personnel in written reports
	Use of bottom-of-the page footnotes (obsolete)

instances, however, the writer may choose whichever style is preferred, as long as it is used consistently. Examples of forms used are the American Psychological Association (APA), Campbell, and Turabian. The exact references for these various styles will be found in the bibliography for Chapter 9. Some universities have published their own writing guidelines and require that they be used.

The Dangers of Plagiarism.   Copying the exact words of others without giving credit to the author and getting permission from the author and/or publisher is an unethical and sometimes illegal act. Such a practice is not acceptable for students, practicing nurses, or experienced researchers. The Copyright Act of October 19, 1976, which took effect January 1, 1978, protects the published and unpublished works of authors. The concept of "fair use," however, allows for the limited use of quotations and paraphrasing as long as proper credit is given to the author and publisher. Long quotes, tables, and graphs may be used with the author and publisher's written permission, but this permission may require the payment of a fee. Even if a fee is paid, proper credit must be given.

The Final Report.   After the content has been prepared, the writer is responsible for the final written product. Effective papers require numerous rewritings. It is suggested that the writer prepare several drafts. Having rough drafts typed triple-spaced is very helpful so that they can be edited and revised more easily. An excellent typing job adds to the effectiveness and appearance of the final paper, but it is the writer's ultimate responsibility to proofread the final report for correct content, spelling, and typographical errors. A cover page with title, name, date, and other essential identifying information should be used. The title should also be included on the first page. A sufficient number of headings and subheadings should be used throughout the report for clarity and ease of reading.

Preparing the Report for Publication

After the final written report is complete, the writer should consider the possibility of submitting the report, after rewriting and additional editing, for publication in a national nursing or allied health journal. Beginning writers may want to share this writing venture with an experienced nurse author who can assist them with the process.

The sharing of research ideas and/or studies with others through publication is an essential component of the research process.[4] It is personally rewarding to receive requests for more information about a published report from other nurses throughout the world. The writer should also be aware of the fact that there will be negative and critical responses as well as positive and praising responses when sharing one's ideas and research findings with others in the profession through publication. All of these factors contribute, however, to the professional growth of the individual nurse and nursing.

Selecting a Journal. The writer will first want to select a journal based on the focus of the manuscript.[5] If the manuscript is to be submitted to a research journal, the manuscript should be written in a research format. If, on the other hand, the writer would prefer to concentrate on the conclusions and recommendations of the study, the manuscript should be written in a format more appropriate for a nursing journal, such as *Nursing* or the *American Journal of Nursing*.

In the university setting, publication in a refereed journal (one in which an editorial board of peers reviews the manuscript without knowing the name of the author to evaluate whether or not it is worth publishing) is considered more prestigious than publication in a non-refereed journal (one in which the journal editors decide whether or not to accept a manuscript for publication).[6] A query letter with a topical outline of the manuscript may be sent to the editors of the journal to determine their interest in the content before the paper is submitted. A query letter may save time, but it is not essential.

Manuscript Format. Regardless of where the manuscript is submitted, it should be edited to focus on the intended reader. The format normally used by the journal where the manuscript is to be submitted should also be followed. The writer should study carefully several articles in the journal selected to determine what form and style are used. A formal term paper is not usually appropriate to submit for publication as is until it has been revised and rewritten for publication purposes.[7] The term paper was written with certain guidelines in mind. The manuscript for publication should be written based on the potential readers and the publisher's guidelines.

Tornquist[8] has suggested that the manuscript include the following four basic parts: (1) "Why I Did It" (the problem), (2) "What I Did" (the methods), (3) "What Happened" (the results), and (4) "What It Means" (the conclusions).

THE ORAL REPORT

If an oral research-related report is to be given at a research seminar or symposium, the following suggestions are presented for consideration.

- Proper use of time
- Audience rapport
- Calm approach
- Positive initial impression
- Use of media
- Answering of questions
- Appropriate appearance

Proper Use of Time

It is important to start and stop the presentation on time if the presenter has control over timing. If there are a series of presentations, however, each one may not start on time. Even so, the presenter should stop at the time planned unless adjustments in timing are announced to all because continuing after an assigned time limit ends tends to decrease interest of the audience and impinges on the time of other presenters. It is good to plan ahead and know exactly what can be deleted if time runs short.

Audience Rapport

The presenter can do several things to increase rapport with the audience. Nurses know that direct eye-to-eye contact with patients/clients is an important communication skill. This same skill is important when speaking to a larger group of people. The nurse should use eye-to-eye contact with the audience as much as possible, rotating the eye contact from left to right and front to back of the audience. Speakers who constantly look at their notes, the floor, one side of the room, or the ceiling do not hold the attention of the audience and important content, therefore, may not be heard.

Presenters must also speak in a clear and loud voice so that they can be heard by everyone in the room. If a loudspeaker system is to be used, it should be tested before the session begins.

Calm Approach

It is normal for many people to become anxious when speaking before a large group of people, especially if they have not had much experience doing so. It does not help to tell someone not to be nervous, however. If speakers remember that they know more about the topic than anyone else in the audience because of long-term involvement with the content, it will usually help to decrease apprehension. Also, some relaxation techniques, such as deep breathing immediately prior to speaking, often help. Adequate planning, *complete familiarity* with the content, and practicing the presentation for a friend also will help.

Positive Initial Impression

In writing a paper the first sentence of a paragraph is important because it catches the reader's attention. The same is true for a formal oral presentation. The speaker should go directly into the topic with an interesting content-related comment. A speaker should never start with an apology of any kind, whether related to timing, topic, voice, or media. Most often the speaker is the only person aware of any extenuating circumstances or weaknesses and mentioning them only brings them to the attention of the audience. Neither is an attention-getting joke appropriate as an introduction to the presentation of a professional paper. Later in the presentation humorous incidents related to the study may be appropriate and add to audience interest.

Use of Media

The proper use of media enhances most oral presentations, particularly if statistical data are to be presented. Excellent transparencies and charts can be made very simply by the presenter. Tracing and poster paper as well as colored pencils are relatively inexpensive and can be purchased in most stationery stores. If finances and time are not major problems, colored slides can be made, perhaps with the assistance of a university or hospital media specialist. Graphs, tables, and figures can be used very effectively to enhance presentations as long as they are clear and concise, and contain enough data to stand alone but not so much information that the transparency or slide is overcrowded. Media are of no value (and detract from the presentation) if they cannot be seen or heard by everyone in the room. The presenter should know how to operate the media equipment and try it out in the room to be used for the presentation *before* the audience arrives.

The use of different colors is very helpful and, if transparencies are used, the revealing technique in which a small amount of content is revealed at a time, is quite effective. Orange, red, green, bright blue, brown, and purple are colors that stand out well in a large room. If the presentation is at a poster session at a convention or research symposium, the poster can include more data (such as an abstract or more detailed graphs) because participants will be close enough to the poster to read it. Having available duplicate copies of abstracts of studies is useful if the presenter can arrange to have a sufficient number of copies made. Sometimes multiple copies of abstracts are required by the sponsoring group.

Answering of Questions

Usually a question and answer period is provided at the end of each presentation. This process gives the audience a chance to clarify questions they have regarding methodology, results, or recommendations, for example. The presenter needs to be aware that there are probably experienced researchers in the audience. If questions are asked that point out problems in methodology or possible gaps or errors in statistics, the presenter should welcome and thank the questioner for the suggestions. The presenter should not be overtly hostile toward such questions. The more secure the presenter feels about the content, however, the more welcome are the suggestions. The presenter should think ahead about what possible questions might be asked and prepare for them. One question frequently asked just for interest is *why* the speaker chose a particular problem to study, if that information has not been included in the oral report.

Appropriate Appearance

Traditionally, nurses have been very concerned about their appearance, although during the 1960s and 1970s there was a trend to emphasize the emerging exploration of knowledge and skills in nursing with less emphasis on personal appearance. However, in the 1980s personal appearance is receiving more importance again in nursing as the emphasis on a different kind of professional image begins to emerge.

Although a uniform will not likely be worn by a nurse when giving an oral presentation, except perhaps in a hospital setting, the nurse should be aware of the impression being made, not only for the nurse and the institution represented, but also for the profession of nursing. It should be obvious that a nurse presenting a professional paper will not wear the same type of clothing worn to a party. Being well-groomed will not substitute for a poor presentation, but it often enhances a good presentation.

SUMMARY

The sharing of ideas, problems, and findings is an essential part of the research process. This sharing occurs through the written and oral word. Whether the nurse plans to report on research that has been completed by others, personal ideas about professional problems that need to be studied, or reports of research that have been completed, effective use of the written word and spoken language are essential. Any professional individual must be able to communicate these kinds of reports in an articulate manner.

Types of research-related written reports are: (1) summaries of published research studies, (2) critiques or evaluations of published research studies, (3) statements of problems identified in clinical areas that need to be studied, (4) reviews of literature related to problems to be studied, (5) research proposals, (6) grant proposals, (7) completed research projects, and (8) research abstracts.

Nurses who want to study a problem systematically will need to write a *research proposal* that will describe the problem, purposes, and proposed methodology before beginning the collection of data. After the study is finished, a complete *research report* will be written that will contain analysis of the data, discussion of results, conclusions, and recommendations, including implications for nursing in addition to the information included in the research proposal.

Researchers also have the responsibility to share their findings with other members of the profession through publication in national nursing or related journals and by oral presentations at research seminars and institutes. A clear, succinct, correct writing style is essential. Oral presentations can be improved with experience and the use of techniques that enhance speaker-audience rapport. The proper choice and effective use of media and attention to personal appearance also can enhance oral presentations.

QUESTIONS FOR STUDY AND DISCUSSION

1 Why is it important for professional nurses to be able to speak and write well?
2 Describe *six* types of research-related written reports.
3 What is the purpose of a research proposal?
4 List the essential components of a research proposal.
5 Name *two* published guidelines on writing style.
6 Describe the difference between a refereed and non-refereed journal.
7 How can a nurse speaker increase audience rapport?
8 Discuss how *three* types of media can be used in presenting research reports and/or findings in an oral presentations.

REFERENCES

1 "Steps for Writing a Grant," *Nursing Research News,* Office of Research and Development, College of Nursing, University of Utah, vol. 3, no. 2, 1984.
2 Ellen O. Fuller, "Preparing an Abstract of a Nursing Study," *Nursing Research,* vol. 32, no. 5, 1983, pp. 316–317.
3 Florence S. Downs, "One Red Earring Standing Beneath an Ill Windmill" (editorial), *Nursing Research,* vol. 33, no. 4, 1984, p. 189.
4 Margretta M. Styles, "Why Publish?" *Image: The Journal of Nursing Scholarship,* vol. 10, no. 2, 1978, pp. 28–32.
5 Joanne Comi McCloskey, and Elizabeth Swanson: "Publishing Opportunities for Nurses: A Comparison of 100 Journals," *Image: The Journal of Nursing Scholarship,* vol. 14, no. 2, 1982, pp. 50–56.
6 Bonnie C. Clayton, and Kathleen Boyle, "The Refereed Journal: Prestige in Professional Publication," *Nursing Outlook,* vol. 29, no. 9, 1981, pp. 531–534.
7 Edith P. Lewis, "The Term Paper," *Nursing Outlook* (editorial), vol. 25, no. 11, 1977, p. 691.
8 Elizabeth M. Tornquist, "Strategies for Publishing Research," *Nursing Outlook,* vol. 31, no. 3, 1983, pp. 180–183.

BIBLIOGRAPHY

Bernstein, Theodore M., *The Careful Writer,* Atheneum, New York, 1973.
Campbell, William Giles, *Form and Style in Thesis Writing,* Houghton Mifflin, Boston, 1954.
Corder, Jim W., *Contemporary Writing,* 2d ed., Scott, Foresman, Glenville, Illinois, 1983.
Day, Robert A., *How to Write and Publish a Scientific Paper,* 2d ed., ISI Press, Philadelphia, 1983.
Fernald, James C., *Funk and Wagnalls Standard Handbook of Synonyms, Antonyms, and Prepositions,* Funk and Wagnalls, New York, 1947.
Geach, Barbara, "People Write Funny Things," *Nursing Outlook,* vol. 26, no. 6, 1978, p. 370.
Goldensohn, Ellen, "Acute Fulminating Jargonitis," *Nursing Outlook,* vol. 30, no. 9, 1982, p. 541.

Kolin, Philip, and Janeen L. Kolin, *Professional Writing for Nurses,* Mosby, St. Louis, 1980.

Mawson, C. O. Sylvester, *Dictionary of Foreign Terms,* 2d ed., Crowell, New York, 1975.

Publication Manual of the American Psychological Association, 3d ed. American Psychological Association, Washington, D.C., 1983.

Sexton, Dorothy L., "Developing Skills in Grant Writing," *Nursing Outlook,* vol. 30, no. 1, 1982, pp. 31–38.

Sexton, Dorothy L., "Presentation of Research Findings: The Poster Session," *Nursing Research,* vol. 33, no. 6, 1984, pp. 374–376.

Turabian, Kate L., *A Manual for Writers,* 4th ed., University of Chicago Press, Chicago, 1973.

RESEARCH IN THE CLINICAL SETTING

CHAPTER 10

APPLYING RESEARCH IN THE CLINICAL SETTING

The emphasis that has been placed on research in nursing over the past several years is apparent. The number of publications that include research reports and research-related activities has increased. Baccalaureate nursing programs have adjusted their curriculums to expand the scope and depth of research content. National nursing organizations have directed their attention toward presentations that reflect the research process and research findings. Currently, leaders in nursing are discussing the need for national nursing research centers where direct sources of funds would be available to nurse researchers. Despite this emphasis upon research and related research activities, the utilization of research findings by those who are in direct contact with patients/clients has been and continues to be minimal.[1,2]

The reasons cited for the limited use of research findings by those in direct contact with patients/clients are varied. Some authors believe the limited use of research findings is due to inadequate educational preparation.[3] Other authors suggest that the limited use of research findings is related to unavailable sources of research or the practicing nurses' unawareness of the research literature.[4] Additionally, some authors suggest that the limited use of research findings is because of poor communication between nurse researchers and the practice community.[5] Although the reasons for the limited use of research are varied, there is little doubt that if an improved image of nursing is to be achieved and the quality of patient care improved, the utilization of research findings is imperative.[6] The purpose of this chapter is to describe the process of implementing research findings in clinical practice, discuss the criteria by which research studies are assessed for implementation, and examine the various ways that research findings can be disseminated and shared.

PRACTICE PRIORITY

The practicing professional nurse has innumerable responsibilities. One major responsibility of today's nurse is that of being a consumer of research. A consumer of research is a practicing professional nurse who consistently reviews the current literature in an effort to ascertain the latest developments on a problem in a selected area of practice. To be a consumer of research, the nurse uses the results of research studies rather than being directly involved in the conduct of research. Conduct of research is directed toward the production of knowledge that is generalizable beyond the population being studied.[7] Research utilization, in contrast, is focused upon the transfer of specific research-based knowledge to clinical practice.[8] For the remainder of this chapter, the terms *practicing professional nurse* and *consumer of research* will be used interchangeably.

PROBLEM IDENTIFICATION AS A CONSUMER OF RESEARCH

In Chapter 3, the identification of researchable problems was discussed. Cues to researchable problems were presented to provide the beginning researcher an idea of how researchable problems are conceptualized. Although the identification of researchable problems and cues to research problem conceptualization are directly related to research *conduct,* many problems that need solutions and many questions that need answers are readily apparent to the practicing professional nurse. Frequently these questions and problems have already been examined through the research process. Therefore, prior to developing a research proposal and implementing the research study, the *consumer* of research begins a search to determine the availability of completed research studies that relate directly to the question or problem under consideration. This search is referred to as the *process of research utilization* and is shown in Figure 10–1.

The practitioner of professional nursing as a consumer of research is not only expected to review the literature on a consistent basis but also to be continually aware of problems and questions developed from the ongoing activities of everyday practice. An awareness of the problems and questions that require solution through research is a *key* to the professional practitioner's utilization of research. Problems or questions identified in the clinical area are derived from several sources, such as patients/clients, peers or colleagues, nursing care activities, and interdisciplinary approaches. In addition to sources in the clinical area, reading the literature and attending conferences that relate to the practitioner's area of practice are viable sources from which research problems or questions concerning nursing practice can be identified and explored. Examples of several problem areas according to their respective specialty that have and continue to be prime areas for research utilization are shown in Table 10–1.

Although the identification of problems and questions may develop from several sources, the major concern of the consumer of research during the problem identification phase of research utilization is to be able to articulate the problem/question in a succinct manner. The problem/question must be able to be communicated by the consumer of research in a clear, concise way.

Problem/question identification	Exploration available studies	Applicability	Implementation assessment	Evaluation	Dissemination of findings
→	→	→	→	→	→
Clear Concise Comprehensive Communicable	Previous studies review Current literature review Peer contact Expert consultation	General evaluation Areas for evaluation emphasis	Fit Sample Environment Professional basis Theoretical merit Relevance to practice Significance Replication potential	Adoption Rejection Modification	In-service education Conferences Publications Continuing education

FIGURE 10–1
The process of research utilization.

TABLE 10–1
SELECTED LIST OF PROBLEM AREAS THAT HAVE BEEN RESEARCHED

Medical-Surgical	Community-Mental Health	Maternal Child	Social, Behavioral, Other
Mobility and dominance	Life events and suicide	Parent-child communication	Nursing roles
Patients'-spouses' perceptions of myocardial infarction	Movement therapy and the aged	Lamaze	Adolescents' perception
Oral temperatures, relations and techniques	Problematic behavior perceptions	Maternal and child attachment	Self-concept, self-esteem
	Consumer participation	Fathers' role in birthing	Body image
Diet temperature	Human sexuality counseling	Labor	Socialization
Decubitus	Community health programs	Single-parent families	Role theory
High-risk appraisal	Life events scaling	Childbirth preparation	Collaborative research
Rehabilitation	Denver Developmental Screening	Pregnancy risks	Compliance
Postsurgical coping	Health risk appraisals	Parental attitudes	Anxiety
Decision-making for surgical in-tervention	Hospice movement	Childrens' locus of control	Death and dying
	Family nurse practitioners and com-munity health	Vaginal and cesarean births	Levels of nursing education
Physiological indices of stress		Breastfeeding	Social supports
Clinical pain	Independent practice	Touch	Nursing process
Preoperative teaching	Institutionalized elderly	Rooming-in	Primary nursing
Hypertension and culture	Risk-reduction behavior	Supportive behaviors in labor	Continuing education
Teaching and compliance	Breast cancer beliefs	Stress and premature labor	Coping
Catheter care techniques	Rape	Environmental effects on preg-nancy-induced hypertension	Depression
Chronic illness	Crisis intervention	Supportive positions in labor	Teaching techniques
Nursing activities and mixed venous oxygen saturation	Discharge planning		Assessing job performance
	Psychiatric nurses' perceptions		Folk healing practices
Intracranial pressure and effects of touch	Well elderly and community re-sources		Evaluation

AVAILABILITY OF RESEARCH STUDIES FOR UTILIZATION

Once the problem/question has been well-developed, several avenues are open to the consumer to determine the availability of research studies. These avenues include peer contact, literature reviews, and the use of experts.

Peer Contact

The use of peers in locating available research studies that are directly related to patient/client care or nursing activities cannot be overemphasized. Through the contact with peers new and frequently different sources of research studies or their findings may be obtained that enable consumers to broaden their perspective and deepen their understanding of the identified problem. As a result of this sharing of concerns and problems with colleagues and peers, additional questions arise that impact upon the identified problem and subsequently suggest new and different ways of perceiving the problem or gaining solutions.

Literature Review

The literature review may involve a number of different approaches. These approaches involve the consumer's ongoing review of current periodicals or publications that are directly related to the identified problem/question. Also, exploration of publications during the past few years is indicated. Frequently the problem is addressed in publications that are not specifically related to the practitioner's area of interest and thus, publications that peripherally relate to the problem also need to be reviewed. For example, if the consumer of research has identified a problem related to care of the patient who has had a stroke, the publications indicated for review would be the *Journal of Neurosurgical Nursing, Journal of Neuroscience,* and the *Journal of Neurology.* Publications that also might be reviewed for stroke-related research include the *Journal of Rehabilitation,* the *Journal of Chronic Illness,* and publications of the American Heart Association. The results of research in all of these journals are becoming increasingly visible. These publications are frequently found in the medical library where the practitioner is employed. Personnel in the employee's medical library are frequently able to assist the consumer of research in obtaining references that are directly related to the problem under investigation. Some medical libraries utilize volunteers to assist in the identification, and more importantly the retrieval, of various publications or periodicals that are needed by the consumers in their exploration of available research findings.

Although the medical library where the consumer is employed is readily available, the selection of library materials is sometimes limited. The use of a library associated with the nearest college or university, therefore, is indicated to review the available literature that relates to the problem under investigation. Various computer searches that were discussed in Chapter 4 further assist the consumer in locating pertinent research references.

Use of Experts

In most areas of nursing practice someone can be found in the consumer's environment who possesses additional education or experience. These individuals are frequently able to provide the consumer of research with information pertaining to the latest developments in a particular area of practice as well as current research findings. Faculty members of the community college or nearby university are also a valuable source of research findings and recent developments in a selected area of nursing practice. If a faculty member from the local college or nearby university supervises students at the consumer's place of employment, contact with this individual is often all that is necessary to find out about pertinent research studies. A telephone call to the college or university dean or department chairperson is also helpful in identifying faculty who may assist the consumer in locating appropriate research references.

APPLICABILITY OF RESEARCH FINDINGS

Once the consumer has reviewed the research studies and their findings from the literature and explored the problem/question with colleagues and those with the appropriate expertise, the consumer is ready to assess a particular study's findings for use in the clinical setting. The assessment involves a systematic appraisal by the consumer of the applicability of the research findings to the clinical practice setting. The assessment must, therefore, involve an evaluation or critique of each of the steps of the research process in order to ascertain the appropriateness of the findings in relation to the consumer's stated research question. The process of reading and evaluating research studies may be found in Chapter 8.

Although the research study is evaluated in its entirety, a number of areas of the research process need particular attention when the practitioner plans to utilize research findings from various research studies.[9] These areas of the research study that need particular emphasis are: (1) the purpose, (2) the assumptions and limitations of the study, (3) the research question and hypothesis if indicated, (4) the methodology, (5) data analysis, and (6) the findings and conclusions. The consumer of research is, therefore, advised to consider the following questions in relation to the particular areas of the research study that need emphasis:

Purpose

• What is the reason the research study was conducted?
• Does the purpose of the research study approximate the consumer's quest for answers?

Assumptions-limitations

• Are the assumptions and limitations of the research study delineated?
• Do the assumptions and limitations of the research study approximate the consumer's situation?

Research question and hypotheses

• Does the research study's question coincide with the consumer's question/problem?
• Is the research question clear, concise, and not open to misinterpretation?

- Are the variables of the research question the same, similar, or different from those under investigation by the consumer?
  - Does the research study's hypothesis predict a relationship between the variables?
  - Does the hypothesis derive directly from the research problem/question?

Methodology

- Is the methodological approach appropriate to the question being asked?
- Is the methodological approach conducive to replication in the consumer's area of practice?
- Have all the factors inherent in the methodological approach been addressed?

Data analysis (consultation may be needed—see Chapter 7)

- Is the means of analyzing the data appropriate?
- Does the data analysis support the answer(s) to the research question(s)?

Findings-conclusion

- Are the findings of the study appropriate to the research question asked?
- Do the findings of the study provide a reasonable solution to the consumer's question or problem?
- Are the findings generalizable?
- Are the conclusions derived and supported by the study's findings?

In addition to the above questions that the consumer is advised to emphasize in the evaluation of the research study, the overall positive and negative attributes of the study need to be assessed. The consumer will, also, need to determine if the study has replication potential because research findings from one particular research study are not subject to generalizability.[10]

IMPLEMENTATION ASSESSMENT

After the consumer of research has determined the applicability of the research study for use in the clinical setting, an assessment of the study's potential for implementation is indicated. This implementation assessment involves serious consideration of the research study's fit, professional basis, and relevance to practice.

Fit

The fit of the research study refers to the characteristics of the sample and the setting in relation to the consumer's sample and setting. Both the sample and the setting require a comprehensive analysis.

Sample.   The sample used in the research study must be assessed in relation to the clients/patients to whom the research findings will be applied. The consumer of research, therefore, will need to determine if the demographic characteristics of the sample in the research study approximate those of the consumer's clients/patients. This approximation includes the following factors:

- Age
- Socioeconomic background
- Educational level
- Diagnosis or type of illness
- Acuity or chronicity of illness

Each of the above characteristics of the research study's sample and the consumer's sample need to be determined and compared. This comparison is necessary to determine similarities and differences of the two groups. If the groups vary to a significant degree the research findings will have limited application. For example, the perception of the quality of life may be considerably different for one group of patients/clients who have recently become ill when compared to patients/clients who have been chronically ill. In addition, dissimilar characteristics of the two clients/patients groups will affect the outcome of the variables.

Setting.   The setting in which the research study was conducted is also a consideration of *fit*. Fit with the research study's setting refers to the environmental factors which if substantially different from the consumer's setting will alter the findings. The findings would thus be inappropriate for application. Factors of the research study's setting that require assessment by the consumer are the following:

- Geographical location
- Kind of agency
- Type of organization
- Time of implementation
- Specific area of implementation
- Timeliness of the study

Each of these environmental factors can influence the findings of the research study if an approximate similarity does not exist. For example, the results of a client/patient medication compliance study may be entirely different for a Veterans Administration Hospital and a county hospital. Also, the findings from a 1970 discharge planning program for postmyocardial infarction patients may be inappropriate for today's consumer's use.

Professional Basis

The professional basis of a research study will need to be considered by the consumer of research. The professional basis of a study refers to its theoretical or scientific merit and the relevance of the study to clinical practice. Each component of the research study's professional basis needs to be evaluated to determine if the findings of the research study are appropriate for implementation.

Theoretical Merit.   Theoretical merit refers to the conceptual attributes of a research study and involves two interrelated factors. The first of these two factors relates to how the research study was developed; the second factor refers to the consumers' bases for practice. How the research study was developed involves the interrelationship between the theories, concepts, propositions, and facts as they support and provide direction to the research question. The theoretical or conceptual basis of the research study being reviewed must, therefore, be assessed according to its soundness or scientific underpinnings.[11]

The second factor of theoretical merit of a research study is related to the consumer's framework for practice. Professional practice implies that the practitioner of nursing provides quality care based on an identified theoretical or conceptual framework. The way the nurse practices, therefore, is not derived from authority, supposition, trial and error methods, or intuition. Thus, interventions by the practitioner are supported by a scientific basis of practice. If the conceptual framework of the research study is in opposition to the consumer's conceptual basis for practice the study's findings would not warrant utilization.[12] However, if the consumer is not currently practicing from a conceptual base, the utilization of the findings from the research study could provide a beginning conceptual base for practice. The consumer's use of the study's findings would, of course, imply that the consumer can comprehend the conceptual base and be comfortable using it as a framework for practice.

Relevance to Practice

Professional significance.   Relevance to practice infers that the findings of the research study are significant to professional practice and implementation is feasible through replication. At times, the consumer of research will determine that the scientific merit of a study is noteworthy and the results of the critique or evaluation positive, yet the study's relevance to clinical practice is minimal. The research findings must be perceived by the consumer of research as having an impact upon the quality of care being provided to the client/patient. The findings must also be consistent with the consumer's initially conceived problem or question. In addition, the findings must be viewed as significant by the nursing community. The question, therefore, that must be asked by the consumer is, "Does this research provide an overall contribution to nursing knowledge?"

Replication potential.   Research findings are not definite, absolute, or generalizable to all settings.[13] The findings from one research study are insufficient to substantiate a change in practice. If a synthesis of two or more studies, however, forms a research base for the proposed change, the findings may provide the necessary evidence for change. A research base is a synthesis of the knowledge resulting from several studies whose findings corroborate, extend, or delineate the concept(s) investigated in the studies.[14] Currently, the research base for problems/questions in clinical nursing is extremely limited. If the findings of only one study are available, the consumer of research should replicate the research study prior to applying the study's findings. This replication of the research study by the consumer is required because the validity of the findings for the consumer's setting must be ascertained. Considerations that need to be addressed include the constraints of the setting, ethical and legal concerns, patient/client risks, personnel support, and the incidental factors of time, money, and equipment.

Constraints of the setting refer to the policies and rules that govern the overall functioning of the institution. Standing policies dictate whether or not different activities or new procedures may be implemented. Standing policies also prevent the utilization of research findings until such findings have been scientifically proven and indicate a need for change. The consumer of research, therefore, will need administrative approval for the replication of the study. The replication of the study may also require approval by the institution's research committee. The consumer of research needs to be aware that institutional policies and rules may impede the process of replication. However, despite the time that may be required to approve the research study's replication, the replication may provide the necessary evidence required to enact change.

Ethical and legal risks are a prime consideration in replicating a research study. Since the consumers of research are obligated to practice according to their respective states' nurse practice acts and provide care according to the act's parameters, replication of research studies frequently carries a legal and ethical risk. The best means to assure that ethical and legal considerations have been met is to obtain appropriate sanction through administrative personnel or the institution's research approval body.

No single research study can provide the necessary valid evidence to justify its use with the recipients of health care.[15] Consumers of research need to be aware of the potential risks patients/clients may be subject to with the implementation of the replicated research study. Clients/patients have rights and they must be consciously observed by the consumer of research. Informed consent by patients is, thus, a prerequisite to replicating research studies. The replication of the research study is no different than the conduct of the research study in the clinical practice setting.

Personnel support is another consideration the consumer of research must acknowledge. Personnel support refers to not only those individuals who serve in an administrative capacity but also to those individuals who are the research consumers' coworkers and peers. Replication of the research study requires the endorsement and the support of all employees of the health care institution who will be directly or indirectly involved. The consideration of personnel support is often neglected by the consumer of research when replication of research studies is implemented. Cooperation of all levels of personnel is imperative to ensure the success of the research study's replication.

The time, finances, and equipment needed to replicate a research study are frequently overlooked by the consumer of research. However, the amount of time involved, the financial assistance needed, and the required equipment to replicate the research study must be considered. Each of these considerations must be assessed from a realistic perspective prior to replicating the research study and planned for accordingly.

EVALUATION

Once the study has been replicated and the findings determined, an evaluation is indicated to determine the value and potential for implementing the research findings. This evaluation involves a decision to adopt, reject, or modify the research findings. If the findings of the replication study approximate the research study's findings, the decision to adopt or accept the findings for implementation in the clinical setting will be favorable. The decision to adopt the findings, however, will depend upon the extent to which adoption of the findings affects the institution. If the decision to adopt the findings relates only to the consumer's primary area of practice, implementation may not cause any difficulty. If the findings, however, have implications for a major widespread change, the decision to adopt will involve acceptance by the entire institution.

If the findings of the replication study are inconsistent with the research study's findings, the decision to reject the findings will be forthcoming. The consumer, therefore, would not use the findings in the practice setting. Different findings from the replication study may, however, simply require that a modification be made in order to implement the findings. Thus, the consumer needs to reassess the findings from the replication study to ensure that the research study's findings are not prematurely rejected. The consumer's decision to adopt, reject, or modify the research study's findings will depend upon the predetermined fit, the theoretical basis of practice, the feasibility of implementation, and a review of the supporting evidence.[16]

Adoption of the research findings does not necessarily end the need for continued evaluation once the research findings have been implemented. Therefore, an evaluation to determine the effects of the implementation of the research findings is indicated. Evaluation tools to assess the findings will need to be developed. To ensure that the change resulting from implementing the research findings does not extend beyond the limits of the research study, the consumer of research must be able to evaluate clinically the effects of the research findings.[17]

DISSEMINATION OF THE RESEARCH FINDINGS

Dissemination of the research findings from replication studies is imperative. Dissemination or sharing of the findings provides the means by which other consumers of research may implement change, based on scientific inquiry, in their respective clinical settings.[18] The dissemination of research findings may assume many forms such as in-service education programs, conferences, publications, or continuing education offerings. The form that the consumer of research chooses to disseminate the results of the replicated research study is not as significant as the fact that sharing occurs.

In-Service Education Programs

In-service education programs provide the means of sharing the replication studies with those individuals who have perhaps been the most interested and involved. Presentations, therefore, to personnel of the immediate environment is highly recommended. If the findings suggest a major change that affects the majority of personnel the presentation of the findings will be essential. If, however, the findings indicate a more localized change, the sharing or dissemination of the research and the findings from the replication study may not necessarily involve all personnel. Success or failure of implementing the research findings, however, necessitates the involvement of all personnel who will be directly affected.

Conferences

Dissemination of findings may be done through various conferences at the local, regional, and national level. This form of sharing allows other professional practitioners an opportunity to learn of research findings that may contribute to their scientific base of practice and improve the quality of care their patients/clients receive. The sharing of replication studies frequently substantiates the significance of the original research study and supports to a greater degree the validity of the findings for scientifically based nursing practice.

Publications

Publishing the results of replicated research studies by the consumer of research provides another avenue that can facilitate change in professional nursing practice. Publishing results of replication studies in refereed journals ensures a wider dissemination of research findings to practitioners, educators, and other nurse researchers. Publication also provides the opportunity for other consumers of research to analyze the findings through written communication and subsequently to evaluate the current status of a particular clinical problem/question. Publishing the findings from replication studies, however, requires that the consumer of research have acceptable writing skills to ensure reader comprehension and meaningful sharing. At times, writing for publication can cause the consumer of research some concern. This concern can be alleviated by attending writing workshops or consulting with individuals who have had favorable results from the publishing experience.

Continuing Education Programs

Continuing education programs provide another avenue of disseminating the results of replication studies. Although continuing education programs may not involve the widespread sharing offered by publications, the participants in attendance are usually highly motivated to learn of new developments in a particular area of practice. Many states have mandatory continuing education requirements and, thus, this avenue of sharing the results of replication studies is usually well attended. The time allotted to present research findings through continuing education programs is frequently limited and, therefore, the consumer of research must be able to share the major steps of the research process and the findings in a well-articulated but abbreviated manner.

SUMMARY

One of the major responsibilities of the nurse today is being a consumer of research, which involves the application of research-based knowledge to clinical practice. The application of research knowledge to clinical practice requires the consumer of research to evaluate a research study through an assessment process referred to as the *process of research utilization*. The process of research utilization begins with a clearly defined statement of the consumer's identified problem or question. A search by the consumer to discover available research studies and their findings involves the use of colleagues, literature reviews, and consultation with experts in the consumer's respective area of interest. An evaluation of the entire research study and specific areas for evaluation emphasis is subsequently implemented to determine the applicability of the research study to the consumer's problem or question under investigation.

After the applicability of the research study is evaluated by the consumer of research, an implementation assessment is indicated. This assessment includes a determination of the research study's fit, professional basis, and relevance to practice. The fit of the research study refers to the characteristics of the sample and setting in relation to an approximation with the consumer's sample and setting characteristics. Professional basis of the research study is assessed according to the study's theoretical merit and its relevance to clinical practice. Assessing relevance to practice involves consideration of two components. The two components of the research study's relevance to practice are the significance of the study to the knowledge base of nursing practice and the research study's potential for replication. An evaluation of the implementation assessment results in the consumer's decision to adopt, reject, or modify the findings of the research study.

The dissemination or sharing of the results of the consumer's use of research findings is imperative. Dissemination of the results may be accomplished through in-service education programs, conferences, publications, or continuing education programs. The form in which the consumer of research chooses to share the results is not as important as the fact that results are shared.

QUESTIONS FOR STUDY AND DISCUSSION

1 Differentiate the terms *research conduct* and *research utilization.*

2 Explain the value of research utilization in clinical practice.

3 Describe the first step in the process of research utilization.

4 Discuss the term *consumer of research* and its relation to professional nursing practice.

5 Name three resources the consumer of research may use in exploring the identified problem/question.

6 Describe the process for evaluating research studies for utilization in clinical practice.

7 Explain the significance of *fit* in utilizing research findings in clinical practice.

8 Discuss the theoretical merit in determining the applicability of research findings.

9 Identify two major components of assessing research findings for implementation.

10 Explain the need for replication of the research study prior to the use of the research findings in the clinical setting.

11 Describe the decision options used in the evaluation of implementing research findings to clinical practice.

12 Name at least three ways that the results of replicated research studies may be shared or disseminated.

REFERENCES

1 James E. Stokes, "Utilization of Research Findings by Staff Nurses," in Sydney D. Krampitz and Natalie Pavlovich (eds.), *Readings for Nursing Research,* Mosby, St. Louis, 1981, pp. 227–233.

2 Jean R. Miller, and Susan R. Messenger, "Obstacles to Applying Research Findings," *American Journal of Nursing,* vol. 78, no. 4, 1978, pp. 632–634.

3 Shirley A. Smoyak, "Is Practice Responding to Research?" *American Journal of Nursing,* vol. 76, no. 7, 1976, pp. 1146–1150.

4 Shake Ketefian, "Application of Selected Nursing Research Findings into Nursing Practice: A Pilot Study," *Nursing Research,* vol. 24, no. 2, 1975, pp. 89–92.

5 Daniel King, Kathryn E. Barnard, and Robert Hoehn, "Disseminating the Results of Nursing Research," *Nursing Outlook,* vol. 29, no. 3, 1981, pp. 164–169.

6 Jacqueline Fawcett, "Another Look at Utilization of Nursing Research," *Image: The Journal of Nursing Scholarship,* vol. 16, no. 2, 1984, pp. 59–62.

7 JoAnne Horsley, Joyce Crane, M. Katherine Crabtree, and D. Jean Wood, *Using Research to Improve Nursing Practice, Conduct and Utilization of Research in Nursing Project,* Grune and Stratton, New York op. cit., 1983, pp. 103–104.

8 Horsley, Crane, Crabtree, and Wood, ibid., p. 104.

9 Ada Jacox, and Patricia Prescott, "Determining a Study's Relevance for Clinical Practice," *American Journal of Nursing,* vol. 78, no. 11, 1978, pp. 1880–1889.

10 Jacqueline Fawcett, "Utilization of Nursing Research Findings," *Image: The Journal of Nursing Scholarship,* vol. 14, no. 2, 1982, pp. 57–59.

11 Fawcett, ibid., p. 57.

12 Cheryl B. Stetler, and Gwen Marram, "Evaluating Research Findings for Applicability in Practice," *Nursing Outlook,* vol. 24, no. 9, 1976, p. 561.

13 Stetler and Marram, ibid., p. 562.

14 Horsley, Crane, Crabtree, and Wood, op. cit., p. 35.

15 Horsley, Crane, Crabtree, and Wood, op. cit., p. 104.

16 Stetler and Marram, op. cit., p. 563.

17 Horsley, Crane, Crabtree, and Wood, op. cit., p. 127.

18 King, Barnard, and Hoehn, op. cit., p. 164.

BIBLIOGRAPHY

Brand, Karen Paulsen, and Ida M. Martinson, "Evolution of a Nursing Research Center," *Nursing Outlook,* vol. 24, no. 11, 1976, pp. 704–708.

Castles, Mary Reardon, "A Practitioner's Guide to Utilization of Research Findings," *Journal of Obstetrics and Gynecological Nursing,* vol. 4, no. 1, 1975, pp. 50–53.

Egan, Ellen C., Beverly J. McEldmurry, and Helen M. Jameson, "Practice-Based Research: Assessing Your Department's Readiness," *Journal of Nursing Administration,* vol. 11, no. 10, 1981, pp. 26–31.

Jacox, Ada, "Nursing Research and the Clinician," *Nursing Outlook,* vol. 22, no. 6, 1974, pp. 382–385.

Ketefian, Shake, "Using Research in Practice: Selected Issues in the Translation of Research to Nursing Practice," *Western Journal of Nursing Research,* vol. 2, no. 1, 1980, pp. 429–431.

Krueger, Janelle C., "Utilization of Nursing Research: The Planning Process," *Journal of Nursing Administration,* vol. 8, no. 1, 1978, pp. 6–9.

Lindeman, Carol A., "Priorities in Clinical Nursing Research," *Nursing Outlook,* vol. 23, no. 11, 1975, pp. 693–698.

Mercer, Ramona T., "Nursing Research: The Bridge to Excellence in Practice," *Image: The Journal of Nursing Scholarship,* vol. 16, no. 2, 1984, p. 47.

Padilla, Geraldine V., "Incorporating Research in a Service Setting," *Journal of Nursing Administration,* vol. 9, no. 1, 1979, pp. 44–49.

Werley, Harriet H., "Research Communication: Impetus to Further Research and Use of Research Findings," *Search,* vol. 5, no. 2, 1982, pp. 1–2.

CHAPTER 11

RESOURCES FOR RESEARCH ENDEAVORS

Research cannot be done in isolation. From the initial development of the research proposal to the analysis of data, resources to facilitate the completion of the research are required. An awareness of the various resources available to the beginning nurse researcher is, therefore, particularly significant. The purpose of this chapter is to describe the subjects, settings, and sources of funding that are available to the nurse researcher in order to facilitate the development, implementation, and conduct of research. In addition, selected ways of organizing research efforts and the identification of significant individuals who can facilitate the research process will be discussed.

SUBJECTS FOR RESEARCH

The well-formulated research question will dictate the type of subjects required for the proposed research. Subjects for research are found in a variety of settings that are concerned with the delivery of comprehensive health care and include the recipients as well as the providers of health care. Subjects for research may, therefore, be patients/clients as well as nurses, interdisciplinary health care providers, and auxiliary health team members. Faculty of schools of nursing and students, in addition, are viable sources of subjects for research. Although more stringent requirements are placed on the inclusion of children and infants in research studies, they too are a source of research subjects.

Based on the research proposed, the number of subjects required to conduct the research may prove problematic. Often, quantitative research studies require a sufficient number of subjects to allow the findings to be statistically analyzed. An adequate number of subjects must, therefore, be identified for inclusion in the research study. Consistent with an adequate number of subjects, similarities among the subjects to promote internal validity must also be considered. In order to obtain a sufficient number of subjects with similar characteristics for the research proposed, more than one setting may be required. The necessity of using more than one setting, however, may alter the research findings due to the inherent differences of the selected settings. The nurse researcher will, thus, need to be cognizant of the number of subjects required and the possible need for more than one setting as well as the potential problems associated with the use of subjects from multiple settings.

Regardless of the number of subjects available for research, informed consent for each subject must be obtained. If children are included as subjects in the research, appropriate means of obtaining informed consent must be determined. Most institutions have developed specific guidelines for obtaining informed consent when children are considered as research subjects. The reader is encouraged to review Chapter 6.

SETTINGS FOR RESEARCH

The settings where subjects may be located for research vary. Subjects may be found in several different settings depending upon the population suggested by the research question. Each setting that is considered by the nurse researcher must be assessed in relation to the availability of subjects and the institution's policies governing the conduct of research. The following are settings where research can be conducted:

- The hospital complex
- Satellite health care centers
- Community settings
  Public health departments
  Extended care facilities
  Public school systems
  Private physicians' offices
  Day care centers
  Group homes
  Industry
- State institutions

The Hospital Complex

The hospital complex includes all of the inpatient units as well as the outpatient and the emergency departments. The majority of completed research studies to date have been conducted in the hospital complex. The hospital complex offers several settings where research can be conducted. These settings include the general medical-surgical units, obstetrics, pediatrics, specialty units, and the operating room. In addition, the outpatient departments or ambulatory care units and the emergency department are settings where research studies may be conducted. Research conducted in these settings can range from the roles and responsibilities of nurses to the care and treatment of patients and clients. Research studies that have used the outpatient or ambulatory care setting have included compliance studies and follow up studies in conjunction with community health agencies and organizations.

Advantages of using the hospital complex as a setting for research are many. Frequently, the hospital complex is the only location where subjects, identified in the proposed research, can be found. Most hospitals also have a research program and a functioning research committee. The hospital, in addition, usually has on staff individuals whose expertise can facilitate the nurse's research efforts. Despite the numerous advantages in using the hospital complex as a setting for research, some disadvantages exist. These disadvantages include the administrative delays associated with research proposal approval, the institution's complex policies governing research, and the need for positive public relations throughout the research process. In addition, priority considerations of routine and diagnostic tests for patients/clients frequently limit the researcher's access to patients/clients.

Satellite Health Care Centers

In addition to the hospital complex, hospitals are currently extending the provision of health care to citizens through satellite health care centers. These centers provide for the treatment of minor emergencies, physical examinations, and health needs of individuals who can be cared for on a walk-in basis. Some of the centers have private sponsors, but many are frequently associated with community hospitals. Most of the centers offer services on a twenty-four-hour basis. Any of the satellite health care centers are excellent settings where nonacutely ill research subjects may be located. Problems that relate to the type of client who uses the satellite center, the incidence of different kinds of health problems, or appropriate nursing interventions in nonemergency health care delivery are examples of researchable studies that can be developed and implemented in the satellite health care center. In addition, questions that involve preventative health care measures can be explored in the satellite centers.

Community Settings

The community offers the nurse researcher a multiplicity of settings for research. These settings include the official local and state agencies of the community as well as private and voluntary agencies. The use of community health care settings for research has been limited in scope, but many of them are viable settings for the selection of research subjects. Access to subjects in these settings is usually feasible. Contact with the appropriate top level administrator in each agency is essential, however, to facilitate implementation of the research according to each agency's policies and procedures.

Most communities publish a listing of their agencies each year. These publications provide the citizen with a guide to available community agencies. The beginning nurse researcher would be wise to obtain such a publication as a resource to identify settings in the community where research can be conducted. The Public Health Department can usually advise the researcher where and how to obtain this publication.

Public Health Departments.   Public Health Departments, particularly those that are considered combined agencies and have a home health care component, are ideal settings where subjects for research can be located. The services offered by public health agencies, such as well-baby and immunization clinics, as well as follow-up services for communicable diseases, provide another resource for research subjects. Screening and case-finding programs also are a valuable resource for research subjects. Public health agencies that are organized to provide home care services in addition are a resource for finding research subjects. These organizations are concerned with the provision of skilled nursing in the home as well as homemaker services provided by home health workers. Occasionally, if skilled nursing services and home health aides are not provided through the official public health agency, Visiting Nurses' Associations and home health agencies may provide the nurse researcher with a source for research subjects.

All health agencies will require administrative approval to conduct research. Nurse researchers who wish to include subjects from the community health agencies will, therefore, be required to have their research studies approved by an appropriate research committee and/or sanctioned by the administration.

Extended Care Facilities.   Extended care facilities provide both skilled and intermediate levels of care to patients/clients. Formerly referred to as nursing homes, these facilities are becoming more significant as the number of older people increases. Although the extended care facility provides care for many patients/clients in the older age category, they also care for patients/clients whose needs do not require hospitalization but a degree of care beyond that available within the home. Thus, patients/clients requiring some degree of nursing care in the rehabilitative stage of illness may be found in extended care facilities. The extended care facility provides a particularly ideal resource of research subjects as the clients/patients found in these facilities reflect some of the more important health care delivery problems facing the nation. The older person who is unable to function independently and the disabled individual recuperating from surgery represent some of the types of patients/clients who are often found in extended care facilities. Problems associated with these situations would be appropriate areas for research conduct. Convalescent and rehabilitative centers are often categorized as extended care facilities.

Public School Systems.   Many public school systems and some private schools are an excellent resource for subjects of research studies. Although health services of school age children are frequently provided under the auspices of the Public Health Department, many areas of the country have a health services component within the public school system. The health services provided by the public school system include nursing, counseling, and guidance as well as speech therapy and hearing evaluation. Since school nurses are involved in screening procedures, case finding, health education, and health counseling, they may be a source of contact for research endeavors.

Private Physicians' Offices.   Physicians in group or independent private practice may provide a resource for research subjects. Since the majority of practicing physicians are specialists in one particular area, their clients/patients reflect health problems consistent with that area of specialization. Research that requires the inclusion of patients/clients with a particular health problem are, therefore, readily accessible. The nurse researcher must get the private physician's written consent to include these patients/clients in the proposed research. The patient's/client's consent to participate in the research must also be secured by the researcher.

Day Care Centers.   Day care centers that include supervised care for both children and older adults is another setting where subjects for research may be found. The use of day care centers for research purposes has received little attention. Day care centers, however, may provide the nurse researcher an ideal setting where research questions may be answered. Research questions that seek answers to the degree of children's well-being without continuous twenty-four-hour parental contact as well as to indexes of quality living for the elderly can appropriately be tested in day care centers.

Group Homes.   The concept of group homes has been well received for several years, yet few researchers consider the group home as a setting in which to seek research subjects. Group homes provide supervised care on a twenty-four-hour basis to the mentally retarded, psychiatrically impaired, foster children, and emotionally handi-capped adolescents and adults.[1] Group homes provide a satisfactory setting where subjects for research can be located and, therefore, researchable questions answered.

Industry.   Many large corporations have a medical or health services department and employ physicians and industrial nurses to provide health care and emergency services to their employees. Programs directed toward health promotion and health maintenance of employees are ongoing services offered by health personnel in industry. In addition, services to employees such as physical examinations, screening for hypertension and heart disease, and dietary instruction and physical fitness counseling are provided. Consistent with the services provided and the number of personnel employed, industry offers the researcher an excellent setting from which subjects may be secured.

State Institutions

In addition to the community agencies discussed above, state institutions also provide a setting where research subjects may be located. State institutions are designed to care for psychiatric patients, the mentally retarded, and prisoners. Individuals confined to institutional care require comprehensive health services and can serve as research subjects. However, due to the stipulations of informed consent in relation to competency and voluntary participation, access to institutionalized subjects for research is extremely limited. The reader is encouraged to review Chapter 6.

FUNDING FOR RESEARCH

Financial assistance to facilitate research conduct is frequently a major concern of the beginning nurse researcher as well as the experienced nurse researcher. To some extent this concern is well-founded, as the process of research involves a number of expenses that are often difficult for the researcher to absorb. Duplication of materials, typing, and instrumentation are a few of the tangible items that may require financial assistance. In addition, expenses for interviewers, observers, and consultants may be needed. Intangible expense items for research include the time and effort expended by the nurse researcher beyond employment responsibilities.

Although many research projects require additional funding that cannot be absorbed by the individual nurse researcher, the type of research indicated by the research question will determine the necessity for funding. Several types of research, such as exploratory, field studies, and case studies, require limited amounts of financial support. In addition, depending upon the research proposed, several of the quasi-experimental research studies, including the nonequivalent pretest-posttest groups, the time series studies, and descriptive studies, can be conducted without large amounts of financial support. Research studies that include large numbers of subjects or require complex instrumentation will, however, necessitate financial support. As the research proposal is being developed, the researcher will be able to determine if funding for the research is needed. Frequently, consultation with experienced researchers will confirm the need for funding.

Beginning nurse researchers are sometimes at a disadvantage when funding for their research is indicated. This disadvantage is due to the inexperience of the beginning nurse researcher and the limited record of conducting research that they can document. The ability of nurse researchers to substantiate their research experience in writing is often sufficient for funding agencies to be favorably impressed. The beginning nurse researcher, therefore, needs to realize that initial requests for funding that are not granted does not necessarily imply a poorly conceptualized or developed research study. Wise researchers, however, will consider limiting the scope of their initial research attempts to smaller studies that do not require large amounts of funding. Most experienced researchers who have been granted large sums of money for their research are aware that their accomplishments in research were initially realized through small research projects without the need for large amounts of funds. Once smaller research studies have been successfully conducted, the researcher is then able to document these experiences. The chances of receiving limited amounts of financial support for research are, in addition, greater. Requests for limited financial support may also be directed to more than one source of funding.

Local Sources of Research Funding

Employer. The researcher's employer may be a viable source for research funds. Although in the past employers have had few funds available to support their employees' research, some changes in this situation are being noted across the country. As the emphasis upon clinical nursing research increases, funds for research endeavors are being subsequently budgeted either through the department of nursing services or by general operating expenses. These funds are mostly found in private hospitals or private community agencies. The beginning researcher, however, needs to be aware of this potential source of funding for research.

Community Agencies. Private community agencies that are health oriented are often sources for research funds. Although the funds may be limited, private community agencies may be willing to support the researcher's study if the conceptualized question is related to the community agency's mission and/or health related interests.

Private Business. Funding for research by the *local* private sector has been minimal. However, sometimes private businesses in the community, for purposes of philanthropy, tax deductions, or genuine health-related interests, are willing to support research. Information about whom to contact regarding funding and the accepted procedure are usually found in national funding publications that cite and describe these local businesses. These publications can usually be found in the public library. Leaders in the community may also have access to the names of prominent businesses that are involved in research funding.

National Sources of Research Funding

Sigma Theta Tau. Sigma Theta Tau is the national honor society for nursing, with 65,000 members and 161 chapters located at universities and colleges throughout the United States. Sigma Theta Tau has been involved in funding research for nurses for several years. Funding requests through appropriate application procedures may be directed to the local chapter or national headquarters. Amounts for funding research vary depending upon whether the funding request is directed toward the local chapter or the national headquarters. Sigma Theta Tau has been highly supportive of nursing research in various areas of nursing practice.

American Nurses' Association. The American Nurses' Association is another national nurses' organization that provides funding for research. Through the American Nurses' Foundation thousands of dollars are awarded annually to nurses involved in all types of research. The research proposal with the accompanying application are processed through the national office. Deadline dates for proposal submission are published in the *American Nurse,* the official newspaper of the American Nurses' Association, or may be obtained through the national office in Kansas City, Missouri.

National Institutes of Health, Department of Health and Human Services. The Department of Health and Human Services is a large governmental body that grants funding for continuing education, construction, demonstration, training, and research. This department has been the largest and most visible source of funds related to health.[2] The Department of Health and Human Services and its respective divisions support numerous projects related to their mission. Funding priorities are identified by legislation or internal policy. Priorities for grants are published in the *Federal Register, Capital Commentary,* or *Public Health Reports.* Program announcements are usually sent to schools of nursing, medical centers, and other appropriate institutions. Specific instructions for completing application forms are available from the Department of Health and Human Services.

Health Resources and Services Administration, Division of Nursing.   Grants for funding research are available through the Division of Nursing and include several different types of programs. The Division of Nursing's Research Project Grants, which are the usual and traditional means of funding research, support research projects performed by the named investigator(s) in an area representing the specific interest and competency of the investigator(s). In addition to its Nursing Research Project Grants, the division also sponsors a Nursing Research Program Grant that supports clusters of at least three research studies focused upon a single theme, and a New Investigator Nursing Research Awards program that supports small studies of high quality conducted by new investigators. The Division of Nursing at times will solicit applications for various research support programs that are directed toward the generation of research in a particular area of nursing. An example of a research support program recently offered by the Division was the funding of grants for the purpose of improving the utilization of research in nursing practice, nursing education, and nursing services administration.[3]

Guidelines for submitting research proposals for most of the grant programs offered by the Division of Nursing may be obtained through the national office in Rockville, Maryland. Deadlines for applications are usually cited in the *American Nurse, American Journal of Nursing, Nursing Outlook,* and the *Council of Nurse Researchers* newsletter. Grants awarded by the Division of Nursing entail substantial sums of money and, thus, the grantees are usually experienced nurse researchers who are proposing large research studies.

PUBLICATIONS OF FUNDING SOURCES

The research funding organizations mentioned above represent only a minimal number of the numerous funding sources available to researchers. Sources of funds for all types of research may be public or private and available to both individuals and organizations. Public funds include those from state and federal sources. Private funds are usually those funds that are available from individual donors, foundations, corporations, and national voluntary health organizations.[4] Most funding sources require that an organization be identified as the recipient of the funds they grant. Several annual publications are available to researchers and provide comprehensive listings of all funding sources. Some of these publications list private funding sources and some list public funding sources. Amounts of money available to researchers are also included in the description. Most of the national publications can be found in the public library of the community. National publications, in addition, may be located in the nearby college or university library or the research development office. The following is a list of the more prominent national publications that identify sources for research funding.

• *Directory of Research Grants.*[5] A publication specifically devoted to alerting educators as well as service personnel to more than 2000 grant programs to support research endeavors or educational projects. Recipients of these grants may be individuals or organizations. The list of funding sources is organized by subject area and includes a description of the grant, deadline dates, restrictions or requirements for applicants, and the address and the telephone number of the granting source as well as the average amount of grants. Proposal guidelines are also included.

• *The Foundation Grants Index.*[6] An annual publication that includes cumulative listing of foundation grants. The listing provides access to funding interests of more than 101 major foundations by subject area, geographical focus, types of support, and the types of organizations that frequently receive grants. Grants of $5000 or more are awarded by 465 foundations for a total of over 32,000. This is an independent national service whose purpose is to provide an authoritative source of information on philanthropic giving.

• *Annual Register of Grant Support.*[7] An authoritative reference source of nonrepayable financial support directed toward academicians, researchers, and those individuals in business, civic improvement activities, and social welfare. This publication provides details in relation to grant support of government agencies, public and private foundations, corporations, community trusts, unions, and educational and professional organizations as well as special interest organizations. It includes both private and public foundations.

• *Foundation Grants to Individuals.*[8] A comprehensive listing of 975 private foundations that provide financial assistance to individuals. The publication describes the various purposes for which financial assistance is granted to individuals and provides a bibliography of reference guides to grants other than those made by foundations. Specifications on foundations given by subject area, types of recipients, and geographical location is included to alert the nurse researcher to any particular limitations.

• *Directory of Financial Aids for Women.*[9] A recent addition to the various publications devoted to the identification of funding sources. Exclusively directed toward financial assistance for women, this directory presents more than 1100 references and cross-references concerned with loans, grants, awards, financial institutions, and general financial aid directories. The directory is arranged to include a descriptive list of financial aid designed exclusively for women, a list of women's financial institutions, a list of state sources, an annotated bibliography, and directories listing general financial aid programs, and a set of four indexes. The directory is international in scope and identifies numerous opportunities available for citizens of various countries.

RESEARCH AS A TEAM APPROACH

Due to the time and energy required to conduct research, team approaches are frequently indicated. Two team approaches to conducting research are *cluster research* and *collaborative research*. Both approaches involve the efforts of several individuals, and they are currently being used in nursing with success.

Cluster Research

Cluster research refers to a team approach to research that encompasses the development of two or more research studies that focus upon a single or central theme. Cluster research efforts may, therefore, produce research findings applicable to a central theme, yet a separate but related component is investigated. An example of cluster research might be focused upon the adaptations or adjustments patients/clients are required to make in relation to chronic illness.[10] The central theme of this example would be chronic illness and the separate but related component(s) might include the management of medical regimens, adjustments to daily living, or the control of symptoms. Chronic illness, as a central theme, could include patients/clients who have been diagnosed as having diabetes, arthritis, or any of the neurological impairments. Another example of cluster research might be the effects of different teaching strategies and techniques on the postoperative course of coronary bypass patients. In this example, the single theme is the postoperative course and the separate but related components are the different teaching strategies and techniques. Cluster research offers the beginning nurse researcher an opportunity to develop and conduct research in an area of interest and provides peer support, yet it limits the time and energy frequently associated with individual research studies. Cluster research is a particularly useful team approach to nurse researchers in the same setting.

Collaborative Research

A second type of team approach to research is collaborative research. Collaborative research endeavors pool the resources of a variety of researchers, agencies, scientists, clinicians, and representatives from different disciplines.[11] Several models of collaborative research exist; however, the researcher/clinician or the education/service model is the most frequently used in nursing. The collaborative approach incorporates the strengths of both areas, while overcoming their respective limitations. Thus, the expertise of the researcher usually found in the educational setting can complement the clinician's experience in developing significant clinically related patient/client problems. Additionally, the researcher and clinician can supplement each other's knowledge and skill in developing the research proposal. Collaborative research offers the beginning nurse researcher peer support and the research expertise of the nurse educator.

Collaborative research can be implemented with large- or small-scale research projects. The advantages of collaborative research include the conceptualization of significant problems in nursing practice, collaborative efforts throughout the research process that encourage peer review, and the experience of learning the theoretical aspects of research in relation to implementation in the real world. A disadvantage of collaborative research is the group approach, which requires compatible membership in order to facilitate the research endeavor.[12] Unresolved personality differences thus can compromise the research process.

In addition to cluster and collaborative research efforts, there is the practice of using a number of individuals in the conduct of research, who are sometimes referred to as research associates or research assistants. Research associates or assistants are those individuals who are selected by the principal, or primary, investigator to assist with the many activities required to implement and conduct research. The research associate is frequently viewed as an equal partner in all aspects of the research process with the exception of the finalization of the research proposal and dissemination of the written research report. The research associate is usually referred to as one of the investigators of the research in contrast to the primary investigator who has total responsibility for the entire research process. Research assistants, in contrast to the research associates, are members of the research team but their responsibilities are usually confined to collecting or collating data. Beginning nurse researchers who are developing research may find that the time and effort required to complete their research without assistance is unrealistic. One or more research associates or research assistants may, therefore, provide additional help.

AVAILABILITY OF CONSULTANTS

Consultation on several aspects of the proposed research is often indicated. Consultants for research are those professionals who possess a special knowledge or skill that is needed to facilitate the research process. Usually, the specific competencies that are needed by the beginning nurse researcher relate to appropriate methods, correct statistical tests, interpretation of the findings, and writing skills. The consultants usually needed are, therefore, research experts, statisticians, and grant or proposal writers.

To develop, implement, and conduct research requires an advanced educational background. Although many nurses are currently prepared at the master's level, few have had sufficient experience with research to be considered experts in this field. Doctoral preparation in and of itself does not imply research expertise. The granting of the doctoral degree denotes that the nurse has demonstrated the skills and knowledge required of a beginning researcher. The recipient of the doctoral degree is basically at an initial point toward developing research expertise. Therefore, the nurse researcher who needs the expertise of a research consultant would be wise to request a summary of the consultant's research experiences.

Research consultants are usually found in the college or university; however, they may be located in various health organizations serving in a consulting capacity. The services of research consultants may be needed for specific parts of the research process; however, the consultant should be able to identify problematic areas of the proposed research from assessing the overall development of the research. The beginning researcher is, therefore, advised to determine the availability of a research consultant prior to implementing the research study. Research consultants may not be needed; however, questions that need answers from experts frequently arise and their expertise is often crucial in avoiding serious mistakes throughout the research process.

Consultation with a statistician is often necessary when the beginning nurse researcher is planning to conduct quantitative research studies. A statistician is an expert or specialist in statistics who is qualified to select the appropriate statistical tests or tools appropriate for the analysis of data. Based on the data analysis, the statistician is able to help the researcher make inferences in relation to the findings. Although the use of a statistician may be indicated, many research studies do not involve analysis of data by complex statistical means and, therefore, beginning nurse researchers may be able to analyze their own data.

If funding is needed for the proposed research, the expertise of a grant writer may be necessary. Grant writers are individuals who have acquired the ability to write proposals in a concise but meaningful manner consistent with the expectations of the granting agency.[13] The grant writer, therefore, is experienced with various proposal formats and the criteria that must be addressed in the written proposal. Recently, the nursing profession has recognized the need for more researchers to be knowledgeable in writing grants and has, through various national organizations, sponsored grant writing and grantsmanship workshops. Expertise in writing grants often is a deciding factor in awarding funds to support research.

SUMMARY

The well-formulated research question dictates the type of subjects required to conduct research. Research subjects may be health care providers as well as health care recipients. Settings where research may be conducted include the hospital complex and the community. The conduct of research has been confined mostly to the hospital setting; however, community agencies such as the public health department, extended care facilities, the public school system, and industry are a few of the many community settings where research may be conducted.

Funding for research is often needed to support research endeavors. Both public and private funds are available through several local and national funding organizations. Local funds include the nurse researcher's employer, community agencies, and private businesses. National sources for research funding include Sigma Theta Tau, the American Nurses' Association, National Institutes of Health, and the Health Resources and Services Administration, Division of Nursing.

National publications that identify numerous funding sources for research projects are available to nurse researchers through their local public libraries or nearby college and university libraries. Most of these publications are annual editions and include a comprehensive description of the many public and private funding agencies as well as guidelines for submitting requests for financial assistance to support research.

Research may be implemented and conducted through a team approach as well as individual efforts. Two team approaches currently used in nursing are *cluster* and *collaborative* research. Cluster research involves the development of more than one research study in which a central theme is the focus. Although several collaborative research models exist, the nurse researcher/clinician or the education/service model is mostly used in nursing. Collaborative research employs the expertise of both researcher and clinician in a complementary and supplementary manner. Team approaches to research may have more advantages than research developed by the individual.

The use of consultants is frequently indicated in the development, implementation, and conduct of research. The research expert, the statistician, and the grant writer are the usual consultants required by the nurse researcher.

QUESTIONS FOR STUDY AND DISCUSSION

1 Explain the relationship between the research question and the type of subjects needed for research.

2 Describe four settings that may be used for research in the community.

3 Discuss the reason(s) research studies may need to be funded.

4 Identify three types of research that may not require funding.

5 Describe the national sources of funding that the nurse researcher might utilize.
6 Name two publications that list public and private sources of funding.
7 Compare and contrast cluster and collaborative research approaches.
8 Describe the nurse researcher/clinician model of collaborative research.
9 Discuss the types of consultation frequently needed by the nurse researcher.
10 Explain the value of consultation in the research process.

REFERENCES

1 Kevin L. DeWeaver, "Deinstitutionalization of the Developmentally Disabled," *Social Work,* vol. 28, no. 6, 1983, pp. 435–438.
2 Ruth J. Steele, *An Introduction to Grants and Contracts in Major HEW Health Agencies,* 2d ed., National Health Council, New York, 1978, p. 19.
3 Ruth K. Aladj, "Grants Available from the Division of Nursing," *Council of Nurse Researchers,* vol. 11, no. 1, 1984, p. 3.
4 Dorothy L. Sexton, "Developing Skills in Grant Writing," *Nursing Outlook,* vol. 30, no. 1, 1982, pp. 31–38.
5 William K. Wilson (ed.), *Directory of Research Grants,* Onzy Press, Phoenix, Arizona, 1984, p. xii.
6 Elan Garonzick (ed.), *The Foundation Grants Index,* The Foundation Center, New York, 1984, p. v.
7 ——— 17th ed., *Annual Register of Grant Support,* Marquis Professional Publications, Marquis Who's Who's, Inc., Chicago, 1983–1984, p. iv.
8 Claude Barilleaux (ed.), *Foundation Grants to Individuals,* vol. 28, 4th ed., The Foundation Center, New York, 1984, p. 4.
9 Gail Ann Schlacter, *Directory of Financial Aids for Women,* 2d ed., ABC-CLIO, Santa Barbara, California, 1982, p. ix.
10 Anselm L. Strauss, and Barney C. Glaser, *Chronic Illness and the Quality of Life,* Mosby, St. Louis, 1975, pp. 13–65.
11 Janet L. Engstrom, "University Agency, and Collaborative Models for Nursing Research: An Overview," *Image: The Journal of Nursing Scholarship,* vol. 16, no. 3, 1984, pp. 67–80.
12 Janelle C. Krueger, Allen H. Nelson, and Mary Opal Wolanin, *Nursing Research: Development, Collaboration and Utilization,* Aspen Systems, Germantown, Maryland, 1978, p. 29.
13 Sexton, op. cit., p. 31.

BIBLIOGRAPHY

Archer, Sarah Ellen, "Marketing Public Health Nursing Services," *Nursing Outlook,* vol. 31, no. 6, 1983, pp. 304–309.
Baker, Constance M., "Moving Toward Interdependence," *Nurse Educator,* vol. 6, no. 2, 1981, pp. 27–29.
Bishop, Barbara, "A Case for Collaboration," *Nursing Outlook,* vol. 29, no. 2, 1981, pp. 110–111.
Burgess, Wendy, *Community Health Nursing: Philosophy, Process, and Practice,* Appleton-Century-Crofts, Norwalk, Connecticut, 1983, pp. 83–122.
Clark, Mary Jo Dummer, *Community Nursing: Health Care for Today and Tomorrow,* Reston, Reston, Virginia, 1984, pp. 485–509.

Compos, Ruth G., "Acquiring Foundation Funds," *Journal of Nursing Administration,* vol. 10, no. 17, 1980, pp. 38–42.

Gortner, Susan, "Research Grant Applications," *Nursing Research,* vol. 20, no. 4, 1971, pp. 292–295.

Hinshaw, Ada Sue, Helen C. Chance, and Jan Atwood, "Research in Practice: A Process of Collaboration and Negotiation," *Journal of Nursing Administration,* vol. 11, no. 2, 1981, pp. 33–38.

Perske, Robert, and Martha Perske, *New Life in the Neighborhood,* Parthenon, Nashville, Tennessee, 1980, pp. 59–60.

Styles, Margretta, "Reflections on Collaboration and Unification," *Image: The Journal of Nursing Scholarship,* vol. 16, no. 1, 1984, pp. 21–23.

CHAPTER 12

INITIATING RESEARCH IN
THE CLINICAL SETTING

To initiate research in the clinical area of practice not only requires an understanding of the research process but also an appreciation of the organizational structure of the clinical setting in which the research is to be conducted. Understanding the organizational structure of the clinical setting provides the researcher with an idea of how the proposed research will be received and processed for approval as well as an expectation of potential barriers that may impede the implementation. The purpose of this chapter is to describe the process whereby research may be implemented in the clinical practice setting and to identify areas of the process that require additional attention to ensure a positive outcome.

PROFESSIONAL COMMITMENT

A commitment to professional nursing implies that the nurse not only utilize research findings in practice as a consumer of research, but also become *adept* at formulating researchable problems.[1,2] A commitment to professional nursing also requires that the nurse have a basic understanding of how research can be implemented in the clinical setting.[3,4,5] To initiate research in the clinical practice area and experience this process through its completion requires an appreciation that the time and effort involved is significant and cannot be done simply as a gesture of professionalism. The most experienced researchers realize that conducting research is a major undertaking. However, once the research idea has been conceived, the research question formulated, and the steps of the research process analyzed from a point of anticipated impact upon the selected clinical setting, the proposed research is near the stage of initiation.

THE PROPOSED RESEARCH

Prior to formally initiating the research in the clinical setting, a number of concerns need to be addressed by the researcher. These concerns are consistent with the actual implementation of the proposed research as viewed by the appropriate approving body of the clinical facility where the research is to be conducted. The first concern is the research problem or question. Does the research question meet all the criteria discussed in Chapter 3 of a well-developed researchable question? The criterion of whether or not the research question is significant to nursing practice becomes particularly important.[6] If the research question can be assessed in a positive fashion, the research has the potential of being well received in the practice setting. The researcher, however, must assess the potential significance of the proposed research from the perspective of those persons who represent the practicing community of nurses. Research questions deemed significant by the researcher are not necessarily viewed as significant by those persons employed in the practice setting. The wise nurse researcher will take into account this possibility and seek validation of the potential importance of the proposed research among practicing professionals.

A second concern that needs to be addressed by the researcher is the methodological approach or design of the research. This concern is directly related to the implementation process and reflects the impact the research will have upon the practice setting. Questions the researcher needs to be cognizant of in relation to this concern are:

- How is the research question to be answered?
- What subjects are required?
- How many subjects are needed?
- How will the data be collected and by whom?
- What special kinds of assistance, personnel, or material will be needed?[7]

These questions reflect areas of specific concern by personnel in the clinical setting and require a well–thought-out plan by the researcher. In addition to the specific concerns that need to be addressed by the researcher, several other broad questions warrant consideration prior to formally initiating the proposed research. These questions include the following:

- Is the clinical setting or clinical facility where the research is to be implemented receptive to ongoing research and research-related activities?[8,9]
- Does the projected implementation process pose any particular problematic areas that require additional consideration to avert possible unforeseen impediments?
- Does implementing the research cause the clinical facility any undue strain in relation to patient participation, staff cooperation, or ongoing efficient functioning?
- Is the timetable by which the research is to be conducted adequate to allow all the steps in the research process to be completed, including a report of the findings to the nursing community that is involved?
- Does an analysis of the organizational structure of the clinical facility provide the researcher the necessary direction whereby the proposed research will be received, processed, approved, and facilitated?

If the researcher can respond positively to the above overall questions related to implementation of the research to the clinical setting, the research being proposed has the potential of being approved. The researcher, in addition, will have some indication that the research may be conducted with success.

PREPARING THE PROPOSAL

A research proposal is a written plan of the proposed research (see Chapter 9 for details of the written proposal). The research proposal will, thus, address the steps of the research process. Proposals developed by students in the educational setting frequently involve a greater degree of development than those research proposals prepared for approval by the practice setting in which the research is to be implemented. The reason for the discrepancy in research proposal development between the educational setting and the practice setting is because of the differing expectations of the two settings. Because of the differing expectations, the practice setting frequently develops its own research proposal formats that are more abbreviated or condensed to afford the approving committee an opportunity to review and evaluate several research proposals at or before the designated meeting times. An additional and more important reason for the differences in research proposal expectations between the educational setting and the practice setting are those steps of the research process that are of particular interest to the respective setting. In the educational setting each step of the research process must meet the criteria of depth and breadth to afford the highest level of research proposal development dictated by quality research and the respective educational institutions. The review of the literature and the bibliography are two areas of the educational setting that require greater development. Personnel in the practice setting, although interested in the entire research that is being proposed, are more concerned with how the research will impact upon the patients/clients. Personnel in the practice setting, thus, are highly interested in invasive procedures that are directly related to their patients' well-being. Questions that become highly significant for the practice setting in relation to research implementation are directly related to informed consent, which will be discussed later in this chapter.

CHAIN OF COMMAND IN THE PRACTICE SETTING

If the researcher is an employee of the setting in which the research is to be conducted, knowledge of the organizational structure of the setting and of the key people who can facilitate the initiation and implementation of the research through appropriate channels is not frequently a problem. Usually the researcher who is employed in the setting in which the research is to be conducted is aware of the chain of command and the organizational structure as well as the key people in the organization who can provide direction to the appropriate person, committee chair, or committee that must approve the proposed research. Most clinical facilities have within their organization a research committee, a human investigations committee, or a designated person to whom research proposals are submitted for approval. If such a committee or designate is not identifiable, the hospital administrator or the director of nursing is an appropriate resource person to whom an inquiry about appropriate channeling of the research proposal can be directed. For the implementation of research in nursing the director of nursing is the *most* appropriate resource person.

If the researcher wishes to implement the research in a setting in which he or she is not an employee, the task of proposal approval may pose some problems. These problems may be alleviated by seeking the names of individuals in top level administrative positions. An appointment with one of these persons is imperative in order that contact be made with the practice setting where the research is to be conducted and entry by the researcher facilitated. This contact will also provide an opportunity for the researcher to determine the appropriate individual or committee chairperson to whom the research proposal can be directed for approval. A secondary gain from contact with someone in a top level administration position may be a potential commitment of support to having the research implemented and conducted in that setting as well as a general understanding of the organizational structure. Contact with a top level administrator regarding the research activity, in addition, is a gesture of professional courtesy that is highly recommended.

STRATEGIES AND POTENTIAL BARRIERS

Experience frequently plays a significant role in the success of any endeavor. Experience is, thus, likely to influence the success of initiating and conducting research in the practice setting. Although the beginning researcher may be at a disadvantage in respect to experience, an awareness of some of the strategies and potential barriers of initiating and conducting research in nursing may be of value.[10] The following strategies and potential barriers are, thus, presented to alert the beginning researcher of possible impediments to initiating and conducting the proposed research.

Informed Consent

Informed consent is a major concern of the practice setting or clinical facility in which approval for the proposed research is being sought. The historical significance and the purpose of the informed consent have been previously discussed in Chapter 6; however, additional concerns remain that the beginning researcher needs to be aware of to prevent delays in initiating and conducting the proposed research.

Informed consent must be obtained from each person who participates in research.[11] Although there may be a difference in the format and the criteria of the consent forms that are required by the educational and the practice setting, definite commonalities of content will exist. It is extremely wise for the beginning researcher to obtain a sample of the required consent form from the appropriate research approval body where the research is to be implemented. To provide the nurse researcher with an indication of the significant components that must be included in informed consent the following questions are presented:

• Does the research proposal include informed consent that is written in lay terms to allow the patient/client to freely and with sufficient understanding consent to be a participant?

- Does the informed consent form allow the patient/client to withdraw from the research study at any time?
- Does the informed consent form state that participation in the research study will not affect his or her care?
- Does the informed consent form stipulate whether or not compensation is a part of the patient's/client's participation in the research?
- Does the informed consent state where and how the researcher can be contacted if questions arise?
- Are provisions identified in the consent to afford anonymity?
- Does the informed consent form provide an opportunity for the private physician to affix his or her signature indicating permission and support for the research?
- Is there a designated space for the research participant to sign and date the consent form?
- Is there, in addition, a space for the researcher to affix his or her signature as well as the signature of the supervising faculty member or an institutional witness?

As indicated above, an opportunity for the physician to affix his or her signature to the informed consent form may be necessary. Although the physician's signature is not consistently required on all consent forms, an appropriate place for his or her signature may be included on the consent form if the research participant or patient/client is a private patient. Providing an appropriate place for the physician to affix his or her name to the consent form offers a gesture of courtesy to the physician and indicates to the research participant that participation in the research is supported by the physician. Geographical location and/or institutional policies will determine if this procedure is indicated. The researcher, therefore, needs to be cognizant of which patients/clients may or may not be under the medical care of a private physician. Private patients are frequently admitted to profit-making health care facilities and medical centers. City and county hospitals or health care centers seldom admit private patients unless the medical care that was needed was determined on an emergency basis. University-affiliated health care facilities may admit both private and city or county patients.

Informed consents are required for all patients/clients who will be participating in any research prior to the actual initiation of the research and collection of data. Informed consent serves as some degree of legal protection against any litigation that may involve the practice setting and/or the employees in relation to the patient's/client's participation in the research. Informed consent, in addition, protects the research participant and the researchers. Informed consent, therefore, serves the practice setting, the research participant, and the researcher. All informed consent forms are kept according to the stipulations of the researcher's sponsoring institution. The forms are, thus, kept for a specified amount of time by the educational institution if the researcher is a student or by the employing agency if the researcher is an employee. The researcher should keep duplicates of each consent form.

Based on the significant importance of informed consent, patients/clients who have been asked to participate in the proposed research must be provided sufficient time to review and reflect upon their participation in the research. The beginning nurse researcher who is anxious to begin data collection frequently is remiss in not allowing the potential research participants sufficient time to give their consent. A period of no less than twenty-four hours prior to data collection is indicated to provide the potential participant sufficient time to reflect upon his or her participation in the proposed research. This amount of time also permits the potential research participants to formulate any particular questions that may have arisen in relation to their participation.

Timetable

To develop, initiate, and implement the proposed research requires a written plan by the researcher of the approximate time each step of the research will begin.[12] The development of a timetable or schedule provides the researcher a guide by which the progress of the research endeavor can be gauged. A sample timetable is shown in Chapter 9. Although a timetable is highly recommended from the period of research question formulation to the completion of data analyses, the timetable becomes particularly significant during the initiation and implementation of the proposed research. The significance of the timetable during this period is due to the researcher's inability to predict the occurrence of unforeseen events. Unforeseen events can cause major delays in initiating and implementing the research. Examples of possible delays include the cancellation of a research meeting to approve the researcher's proposal, required revisions of the research proposal that are recommended by the research committee prior to final approval, or an insufficient number of potential research participants. Experienced researchers are well aware of these delays as well as other unforeseen delays that impede the progress of initiating and implementing research. These situations cannot be prevented by the researcher; however, a timetable or schedule that reflects flexibility can help to lessen the impact of unforeseen events and delays. The experienced researcher will develop a flexible timetable to accommodate the occurrence of unforeseen events and sometimes will in addition formulate a timetable consisting of two schedules to allow for the occurrence of unforeseen events.

Public Relations

Acknowledgment of the value of public relations is frequently overlooked by the beginning nurse researcher. Public relations refers to the researcher's ability to initiate and maintain satisfactory interpersonal relationships from the time the idea for research arises to the point of communication of the research findings. Positive public relations can facilitate or impede the entire research process. The practice setting in which the research is to be conducted is a particular public relations concern. Therefore, the beginning nurse researcher needs to be aware of the following considerations in initiating and implementing the proposed research in the practice setting:

- Is the *chain of command* being followed?
- Is the researcher able to articulate the proposed research in a concise and meaningful way to all levels of personnel?
- Are the stipulations of the approved research proposal being closely followed?
- Have all personnel who will be involved or associated with the proposed research been advised?

• Have the conditions under which the research is to be conducted been explained to all personnel?

• Have negotiations been conducted with the appropriate persons in relation to the time and conditions under which the data will be collected?

• Is the research committee being apprised at intervals of the progress of the research?

• Is the researcher easily identified? For example, does the researcher wear a name tag indicating he or she is a member of a particular study group?

• Is the researcher's attire consistent with the practice setting's policies?

The above considerations are applicable to the nurse researcher who is employed in the practice setting, the nurse researcher who may be a student, or the experienced researcher who requests entry to the practice setting to conduct research. Satisfactory public relations is a part of the research process that is under the direct control of the researcher and can significantly influence the process and the outcome of the research.

Realistic Self-Expectations

An understanding of research and the research process as well as a positive attitude toward research is required to initiate and implement research in the practice setting. Problem/question formulation, design selection, and validity and reliability measures as well as data collection and analysis techniques are a few of the essential understandings required to conduct research. How can the beginning nurse researcher cope with these multiple expectations and yet be committed to conducting research in the practice setting? A potential way in which the researcher can meet these expectations is to acknowledge and internalize realistic self-expectations. Thus, the beginning researcher needs to understand that there are means by which the expectations of initiating and conducting research in the practice setting can be met. The means to meet these expectations are the use of collegial support, collaboration between education and nursing service, and consultations with experienced researchers.

Collegial Support. Frequently the ideas for researchable problems and the encouragement to pursue research studies are influenced by the beginning researcher's colleagues or peers. Colleagues or peers often serve as a *sounding board* for the researcher's ideas and subsequently assist in the clarification and/or validation of these ideas. Colleagues or peers are also particularly helpful considering the long time required to initiate and implement research. In addition, colleagues provide a source of ongoing support that may be required during periods of time when problems develop or unforeseen delays occur during the initiation and implementation of the proposed research. Most beginning researchers who have been able to complete their research studies have identified their colleagues or peers as being highly influential in the research process.

Collaboration. A second way in which the beginning researcher can attain all the expectations required to conduct research in the practice setting is by the use of collaboration. Whether the beginning researcher is in the educational setting or the nursing service setting does not negate the need for the expertise of the other setting. Consultation in a collaborative way ensures to a greater extent the quality of the research. Beginning researchers often forget that the goals of nursing education and nursing service are the same.

Consultation. Consultation with experienced nurse researchers offers a third way in which the multiple expectations of the beginning nurse researcher can be met. The beginning nurse researcher must be assertive in locating the experienced nurse researcher for consultation. A university-based school or college of nursing is an appropriate place to locate qualified and experienced nurse researchers. Frequently, a telephone call to the college or school is all that is required to arrange a time for consultation. Another source of experienced nurse researchers are research committee members of the health care institution. Most nurses who have been appointed to research committees of their institution have had some experience in conducting research or have been associated with multiple research activities. Frequently the beginning researcher can consult with nurses associated with university schools or colleges of nursing or staff nurses serving on their institution's research committee.

SUMMARY

A commitment to professional nursing requires that the nurse not only utilize research findings in the practice setting but also be able to formulate researchable problems and initiate small research studies in an attempt to solve problems. Research is a major undertaking and requires that the beginning nurse researcher develop and submit a written proposal to the practice setting where the research is to be conducted. Two concerns of the research that will be of considerable importance to the practice setting are the appropriateness of the research question and the process by which the research will be implemented. Several overall questions that need to be considered by the researcher relate to the organization of the practice setting and the receptivity of research activities.

Research proposals that are required by the educational setting and the practice setting prior to the implementation of the proposed research are frequently different. Commonalities, however, reflected in the two research proposals will exist. Wisdom dictates that the beginning nurse researcher contact the practice setting where the research is to be implemented to ascertain the particular specifications of the research proposal. An appreciation and understanding of the organizational structure in relation to the practice setting's chain of command is important in the facilitation of initiating and implementing the proposed research.

Several strategies for and potential barriers to initiating and implementing research in the practice setting exist and include informed consent, the research timetable, public relations, and realistic self-expectations. To initiate and implement research in the practice setting places a multiple number of expectations on the beginning nurse researcher. Having realistic self-expectations, in conjunction with seeking collegial support, collaboration, and consultation will facilitate the attainment of these expectations.

QUESTIONS FOR STUDY AND DISCUSSION

1 Discuss four areas of the clinical practice setting that require consideration prior to formally initiating the proposed research.

2 Name two specific concerns of the practice setting in relation to implementing research.

3 Describe the purpose of the research proposal.

4 Explain the differing expectations of the educational setting and the practice setting in relation to research proposal development.

5 Analyze the value of the chain of command in the practice setting in relation to initiating a proposed research study.

6 Discuss the significance of informed consent from the perspective of the research participant, the researcher, and the personnel employed in the practice setting.

7 Describe five components of informed consent that must be included in the research participant's consent form.

8 Discuss the measures that may be taken by the nurse researcher to ensure the potential research participant is an informed participant.

9 Explain the term *realistic self-expectations* in relation to the beginning nurse researcher.

10 Identify three strategies to facilitate the initiation and implementation of the proposed research.

REFERENCES

1 Carol Lindeman, and D. Schentz, "The Research Question," *Journal of Nursing Administration,* vol. 10, no. 12, 1982, pp. 6–11.

2 Ellen O. Fuller, "Selecting a Clinical Nursing Problem for Research," *Image: The Journal of Nursing Scholarship,* vol. 29, no. 2, 1982, pp. 60–61.

3 Constance M. Baker, "Moving Toward Interdependence: Collaboration," *Nursing Education,* vol. 6, no. 2, 1981, pp. 27–29.

4 Barbara Bishop, "A Case for Collaboration," *Nursing Outlook,* vol. 29, no. 2, 1981, pp. 110–111.

5 Rona F. Levin, "Research for the Undergraduate: Too Much Too Soon?" *Nursing Outlook,* vol. 31, no. 5, 1983, pp. 258–259.

6 Elaine Larson, "Nursing Research Outside Academia: A Panel Presentation," *Image: The Journal of Nursing Scholarship,* vol. 13, no. 3, 1981, pp. 75–77.

7 Marilyn Oberst, "Nursing Research: New Definitions, Collegial Approaches," *Cancer Nursing,* vol. 3, no. 6, 1980, pp. 459–563.

8 Maxine E. Loomis, and Kathleen P. Krone, "Collaborative Research Development," *Journal of Nursing Administration,* vol. 10, no. 12, 1980, pp. 32–35.

9 Susan B. Steckel, "Facilitation Research: Perceptions of the Staff Nurse," *Reflections,* vol. 8, no. 7, 1982.

10 Nancy C. Sayner, "Research in the Clinical Setting: Potential Barriers to Implementation," *Journal of Neurosurgical Nursing,* vol. 16, no. 5, 1984, pp. 279–281.

11 Ada Sue Hinshaw, Helen C. Chance, and Jan Atwood, "Research in Practice: A Process of Collaboration and Negotiation," *Journal of Nursing Administration,* vol. 11, no. 2, 1981, pp. 33–38.

12 Juanita W. Fleming, "Selecting a Clinical Nursing Problem for Research, *Image: The Journal of Nursing Scholarship,* vol. 16, no. 2, 1984, pp. 62–64.

BIBLIOGRAPHY

Brink, Pamela J., and Marilyn J. Wood, *Basic Steps in Planning Nursing Research, from Question to Proposal,* Wadsworth Health Sciences Division, Monterey, California, 1983.

Dempsey, Patricia Ann, and Arthur D. Dempsey, *The Research Process in Nursing,* Van Nostrand, New York, 1981.

Diers, Donna, *Research in Nursing Practice,* Lippincott, Philadelphia, 1979.

Downs, Florence, *A Source Book of Nursing Research,* Davis, Philadelphia, 1984.

Downs, Florence, and Juanita W. Fleming: *Issues in Nursing Research,* Appleton-Century-Crofts, New York, 1979.

Horsley, Jo Anne, et al., *Using Research to Improve Nursing Practice: A Guide,* Grune and Stratton, New York, 1983.

Krampitz, Sydney, and Natalie Pavlovich, *Readings for Nursing Research,* Mosby, St. Louis, 1981.

Krueger, Janelle C., Allen H. Nelson, and Mary O. Wolanin: *Nursing Research: Development, Collaboration, and Utilization,* Aspen Systems, Germantown, Maryland, 1978.

Notter, Lucille, *Essentials of Nursing Research,* 2d ed., Springer, New York, 1981.

Sweeney, Mary Ann, and Peter Olivieri, *An Introduction to Nursing Research,* Lippincott, Philadelphia, 1981.

Treece, Eleanor W., and James W. Treece, *Elements of Research in Nursing,* Mosby, St. Louis, 1982.

Verhonick, Phyllis J., and Catherine C. Seaman, *Research Methods for Undergraduate Students,* Appleton-Century-Crofts, New York, 1978.

GLOSSARY OF BASIC RESEARCH TERMINOLOGY

abstract. A 150- to 200-word summary of a research report that includes the problem statement, methodology, results, and implications.

accident sample. Convenience sample.

analysis of variance. A statistical procedure which is used to determine if there is a significant difference between three or more sets of data.

chi square. A nonparametric statistical procedure that is used with nominal level data to determine if there is a significant difference between two or more groups in some way.

concept. A one-word image or mental picture of some phenomenon.

content validity. The degree to which the items of an instrument measure the content intended to be measured.

control group. The group of subjects that do not receive the treatment in an experimental study. Data on the control group are used to compare with the experimental group.

convenience sample. A sample of subjects who are chosen simply because they are readily available. Sometimes called an *accidental sample*.

correlation. The way in which two variables are related to each other.

correlation coefficient. A mathematical determination of the degree of relationship between two variables. In a positive correlation, as one variable increases (or decreases), the second variable also increases (or decreases). A perfect positive correlation is $+1.0$. In a negative correlation, as one variable increases, the second variable decreases, or vice versa. A perfect negative correlation is -1.0.

data. Information or facts about specific things, persons, or events.

deductive thinking. Taking statements known to be true and deducing other statements.

dependent variable.   The variable that is acted upon by the independent variable.

descriptive research.   Research that describes the characteristics and frequency of certain events.

descriptive statistics.   Mathematical formulas (such as the mean) that are used to describe specific data.

experimental group.   The group of subjects that receives the treatment or manipulation.

experimental research.   Research in which a specific variable or treatment is tested out or manipulated in one or more ways.

halo effect.   One observation or report is influenced in some way because of a similar observation or report.

Hawthorne effect.   The subjects in a study act or react in a certain way just because they are in a study, thus affecting the results.

hypothesis.   The predicted expected relationship between two variables; a hunch.

independent variable.   The variable that acts upon or changes the dependent variable in some way. The treatment or experiment to be tested.

inductive thinking.   (1) A synthesis of ideas and thoughts in which factors pertaining to a specific phenomenon or situation are conceived and related to other situations. (2) The application of the factors of a specific situation that are generalized to other situations.

interval measurement.   Data points are measured in equidistant quantitative values for a specific factor or characteristic.

mean.   The mathematical average.

median.   The middle number.

mode.   The most frequently occurring number.

null (statistical) hypothesis.   A statistical hypothesis that is stated in the negative form.

nominal measurement.   Measurement of variables that are assigned to mutually exclusive, nonnumerical categories.

ordinal measurement.   Ranking or ordering of a specific category or characteristic.

pilot study.   A preliminary minisimulation of the proposed research.

population.   The total number of subjects who meet the specific criteria for a research study. Sometimes referred to as the *universe.*

primary sources.   Original sources of data or information.

qualitative research.   Research concerned with the collection, collation, and analysis of data that is not amenable to quantification or measurement.

random sample.   The selection of subjects so that each one has an equal chance of being selected.

range.   The difference between the highest and lowest number in a set of numbers.

ratio measurement.   Measurement of factors or characteristics that have a true absolute zero.

reliability.   The degree to which an instrument measures a variable in the same way over a period of time.

research.   The scientific and systematic collection and analysis of data in order to explain events, solve problems, and add to the body of knowledge.

sample.   That portion of the population, or universe, that is selected to participate in a research study.

secondary sources.   Sources of data or information that have been extracted and/or summarized from the original sources.

standard deviation.   The average deviation from the mean.

statistical (null) hypothesis.   A hypothesis that is stated in the negative form.

subject.   A person who participates in a research study.

theory.   The invention of concepts, propositions, assumptions, and facts in a relationship. A proposed systematic set of beliefs, concepts, and/or principles that attempt to explain something but that have not been shown to be true.

universe.   Population.

validity.   The degree to which an instrument measures what it is supposed to measure.

variable.   Any characteristic that changes or varies from time to time.

SAMPLE LIST
OF NURSING JOURNALS

Name of Journal	Subscription Address	Frequency of Publication	Primary Focus
American Journal of Public Health	Publication Sales Division American Public Health Association 1015 15th Street NW Washington DC 20005	Monthly	A general health care journal of particular interest to community health nurses.
Advances in Nursing Science	Aspen Systems Corporation 16792 Oakmount Avenue Gaithersburg, MD 20877	Quarterly	Topics on theory construction, education, nursing philosophy, nursing diagnosis, and nursing research.
American Journal of Nursing	American Journal of Nursing Company 555 West 57th Street New York, NY 10019	Monthly	Articles on all areas of nursing. A few research studies are reported.
AORN Journal	10170 E. Mississippi Avenue Denver, CO 80231	Monthly	Official publication of the Association of Operating Room Nurses. Topics of special interest to the nurse who is interested in operating room nursing.
Critical Care Nurse	Critical Care Nurse, Inc. 680 Route 206 North Bridgewater, NJ 08807	Bimonthly	Clinical articles related to critical care nursing.
Heart and Lung: The Journal of Critical Care	The C. V. Mosby Company 11830 Westline Industrial Drive St. Louis, MO 63146	Bimonthly	Official publication of the American Association of Critical Care Nurses. Articles related to critical care nursing. Some research-related articles are published.
Image: The Journal of Nursing Scholarship	Sigma Theta Tau 1100 Waterway Boulevard Indianapolis, IN 46202	Quarterly	Official journal of Sigma Theta Tau, national honor society in nursing. Publishes research and other scholarly articles.
Issues in Comprehensive Pediatric Nursing	Hemisphere Publishers, Inc. 14 West 44th Street New York, NY 10036	Bimonthly	Topics related to the nursing care of children and adolescents. Articles on theory, research, and practice.

Journal	Publisher	Frequency	Description
Journal of Community Health Nursing	Lawrence Erlbaum Associates, Inc. 365 Broadway Hillsdale, NJ 07642	Quarterly	General articles of interest to the community health nurse.
Journal of Emergency Nursing	C. V. Mosby Company 11830 Westline Industrial Drive St. Louis, MO 63146	Bimonthly	Official publication of the Emergency Department Nurses' Association. A journal of interest to nurses who are employed in the emergency department.
Journal of Gerontological Nursing	Charles B. Slack, Inc. 6900 Grove Road Thorofare, NJ 08086	Monthly	Contains articles related to the care of older adults. Research-related articles are published occasionally.
Journal of Neurosurgical Nursing	428 E. Preston Street Baltimore, MD 21202	Bimonthly	Primarily nursing care articles in the area of neurosurgical and neurological nursing care. Research articles are included.
MCN: The American Journal of Maternal Child Nursing	555 West 57th Street New York, NY 10019	Bimonthly	Articles on a variety of topics related to maternal and child care.
Maternal-Child Nursing Journal	437 Victoria Building 3500 Victoria St. Pittsburgh, PA 15261	Quarterly	Research, literature reviews, and case studies related to mothers and children.
Nursing	Fulfillment Department 1111 Bethlehem Pike Springhouse, PA 19477	Monthly	Topics relating to clinical nursing. No emphasis on research studies.
Nursing and Health Care	Health Science Division Technomic Publishing Company, Inc. 851 New Holland Avenue Box 3535 Lancaster, PA 17604	Monthly (except July and August)	Official publication of the National League for Nursing. Includes a variety of articles on nursing practice, education, and administration.
Nursing Clinics of North America	W. B. Saunders Company West Washington Square Philadelphia, PA 19105	Quarterly	Topics on all areas of nursing practice and nursing education.

Name of Journal	Subscription Address	Frequency of Publication	Primary Focus
Nursing Forum	Nursing Publication, Inc. Box 218 Hillsdale, NJ 07642	Quarterly	A wide variety of topics in all areas of nursing.
Nursing Outlook	American Journal of Nursing Company 555 West 57th Street New York, NY 10019	Monthly	Articles related to all areas of nursing with particular emphasis on education.
Nursing Research	555 West 57th Street New York, NY 10019	Bimonthly	Detailed reports of nursing research, abstracts of nursing studies, and articles on research design and methodology.
Nursing Research Report	American Nurses' Foundation, Inc. 2420 Pershing Road Crown Center Kansas City, MO 64108	Quarterly	Contains information on grants by the American Nurses' Foundation, Inc., research reports and abstracts, and research news.
Pediatric Nursing	Anthony J. Jannetti, Inc. Box 56 North Woodbury Road Pitman, NJ 08071	Bimonthly	Official publication of the National Association of Pediatric Nurse Associates and Practitioners, Inc. Topics on all areas of pediatric nursing. Theoretical and research articles included.
Public Health Nursing	Blackwell Scientific Publications, Inc. 52 Beacon Street Boston, MA 02108	Quarterly	A variety of topics in the area of public health nursing. Includes research articles.
Research in Nursing and Health	20th and Northampton Streets Easton, PA 18042	Quarterly	Research in many areas of nursing and health care.
The Journal of Professional Nursing	American Association of Colleges of Nursing One Dupont Circle Suite 530 Washington DC 20036	Bimonthly	Articles on the practice, research, policy roles, and educational and management concerns of professional nurses.

The Journal of Nursing Administration	2350 Virginia Avenue Hagerstown, MD 21740	11 times per year	Articles on administration in nursing. Generally does not publish complete research studies, although brief research reports are published.
Western Journal of Nursing Research	Western Journal of Nursing Research 1330 South State College Blvd. Anaheim, CA 92806	Quarterly	All topics related to nursing research.

From (1) Warner, Steven D., and Schweer, Kathryn D. (eds.): *Author's Guide to Journals in Nursing and Related Fields*, Haworth, New York, 1982; and (2) Binger, Jane L., and Jensen, Lydia M.: *Lippincott's Guide to Nursing Literature*, Lippincott, Philadelphia, 1980.

SAMPLE LETTER
TO AN AGENCY
TO REQUEST PERMISSION
TO CONDUCT RESEARCH

3300 Fox Glen Lane
Forrest City, California
October 9, 1985

Sally N. Jones, R.N., M.S.N.
Associate Vice President of Nursing
Forrest City General Hospital
Forrest City, California 90000

Dear Ms. Jones:

I am in the process of completing a research proposal and I am currently seeking appropriate clinical facilities where the research can be implemented. The research proposed involves nursing intervention of positioning the patient and its relationship to varying degrees of patient comfort. A copy of the research proposal is enclosed for your review.

I have been advised that prior to any plans to implement my research in Forrest City General Hospital, I must have appropriate administrative approval. Therefore, I am requesting your permission or the approval of the appropriate research committee to proceed with plans for implementing this research at Forrest City General Hospital. Since I believe a meeting may be indicated, I can be located at _____ during the day. If there are any pertinent guidelines to submitting research proposals, I would appreciate it if you would forward a copy to me at the above address.

I look forward to hearing from you, and I appreciate your time in this matter. Thank you.

Sincerely,

Jane M. Doe, R.N.

SAMPLE OF AGENCY'S RESPONSE LETTER AND RESEARCH PROPOSAL REVIEW PROCESS SENT TO RESEARCHER

St. Joseph Hospital
1401 South Main Street
Fort Worth, Texas 76104
Area Code 817 336–9371

January 28, 1985

Dear Investigator:

The Nursing Service Department of St. Joseph Hospital has recently formed a Research and Publication Committee. It will be the function of this committee to evaluate and approve requests for agency participation in research studies that involve nursing staff and/or patients and their families. The focus of the committee will be twofold: (1) to assure the protection of rights of participants in the study, and (2) to address how data collection will be accomplished. The attached will provide useful information regarding how this process proceeds.

Potential studies involving patients/families or staff of St. Joseph Hospital are reviewed at meetings of this committee on the fourth Wednesday of every month. In order for the committee to make the most informed decision possible, we request that you submit, at least two weeks prior to the meeting, two copies of a summary of your study, a copy of your Human Rights Committee approval, your tool, and your agency consent form. This summary will not exceed five pages in length and will include the following: problem of study; theoretical or conceptual framework; hypothesis(es); procedure for collection and treatment of data—setting, population and sample, instruments, data collection, treatment of data.

You are scheduled to meet with the Research and Publication Committee at 10:00 AM on Wednesday, _____. The meeting will take place in 7 Main Conference Room of St. Joseph Hospital. Please be prepared to address the following points at the committee meeting:

a. A brief outline of the background, purpose, and nature of your study.

b. What are the potential risks, and the potential benefits, associated with this study? Who is subject to any risk?

c. How will you communicate regarding risk to potential subjects, or any other involved individuals?

d. What is your procedure for obtaining informed consent?

e. How is your subject selection to take place?

f. How do you intend to protect the confidentiality of your data?

g. Are hospital personnel to be involved in any way in subject selection, data collection, or the processing of data (include picking up questionnaires, etc.)? If yes, how many worker-hours do you anticipate this will involve?

Following the review of your proposal by the committee, one of two things will happen:

a. The committee members will recommend that your study be approved for data collection at St. Joseph Hospital.

b. Recommendations will be made that must be fulfilled prior to another review of your proposal by the committee.

You will be notified of the decision of the committee within two days of the review meeting.

This process is not meant to be cumbersome. It is designed to help you to be ready for review by the Nursing Research and Publication Committee, and to facilitate the involvement of St. Joseph Hospital in the research process.

Good luck to you! Please feel free to call me at 336–9371, extension 5583 if you have any questions.

Sincerely,

Kay Willis, RN, MS
Chairman
Nursing Research and Publication
Committee

ds
Enclosure

DEPARTMENT OF NURSING SERVICE
RESEARCH AND PUBLICATION COMMITTEE

Research Proposal Review Process

Investigator	Agency

---

1. Contacts Agency/Committee for approval for study.

    2. Sends investigator copy of criteria, and letter explaining review process.

       Lists investigator on Agenda of Research and Publication Committee Meeting.

3. Submits the following forms to the Committee at least two weeks prior to its next scheduled meeting:

Two copies of summary of study
Human Rights Approval from "home" agency
Agency Consent Form
Participant Consent Form
Tool

    4. Upon receipt of the forms from the prospective investigator, the Chairperson of the Research and Publication Committee distributes the information to all the members of the Committee for their review prior to the meeting.

5. Meets with the Committee, and briefly presents a general overview of the proposed study. Answers questions raised by Committee members.

    6. Asks questions of prospective investigator.

    7. Informs prospective investigator of the decision of the Research and Publication Committee.

       If approval is granted, signed agency consent form is given to investigator, and one copy retained in the Committee files.

       If approval is not given, recommendations are made to the investigator; who, upon meeting them, may reapply for approval.

    8. Advises any hospital staff that will be involved in the study of the approval of the proposal for research at St. Joseph's.

DEPARTMENT OF NURSING SERVICE
RESEARCH AND PUBLICATION COMMITTEE

Research Proposal Review Process

Investigator	**Agency**
9. Receives approval.	
10. Meets with any involved hospital staff (e.g., head nurse, ADN, or other).	
11. Selects subjects, obtains informed consent, and collects data.	
12. Reports results of research to Agency in writing.	13. Receives report of investigator. Retains report, and all previously submitted documentation in Committee file.

St. Joseph Hospital
Department of Nursing Service
Nursing Research and Publication Committee
Approved: 4/85
Used with permission.

SAMPLE INFORMED CONSENT FORM (CLIENT/PATIENT)

FAMILIAL LONGEVITY PATTERNS AND HEALTH PRACTICES OF PERSONS AGE 85 AND OLDER

I voluntarily agree to answer questions in this interview and understand that I may refuse to answer any question or stop the interview at any time if I desire. I understand that my name will not be recorded or included anywhere in this study except on this consent form, which will be kept separate from the interview form.

I understand that the primary purposes of this study are to determine to what extent long life runs in families, what kinds of health practices contribute most to long life, and what kinds of health problems and health care needs older people have.

I understand that there are no risks or discomforts involved in answering these questions and that there may be benefits to others by determining factors that contribute to long life.

I understand that I may ask questions about the study at any time if I so desire.

_____   _____

Signature of Interviewee   Date

_____   _____

Signature of Investigator   Date

I have read the above information to each person requested to participate in the interview. It is my opinion that each person understands the risks, benefits, and obligations involved in participation in this study (for use when oral consent is necessary because the person cannot see well enough to read or sign the consent form).

_____   _____
Signature of Investigator   Date

_____ has verbally agreed to participate in an interview on familial longevity patterns and health practices.

_____   _____
Witness   Date

SAMPLE INFORMED CONSENT FORM (PERSONNEL)
Texas Christian University

CONSENT TO ACT AS PARTICIPANT IN STUDY OF PERCEIVED AND OPERATIONALIZED NURSING ROLES OF ASSOCIATE DEGREE AND BACCALAUREATE GRADUATES

I agree to have Ms. Debra Glidewell, a senior honors student of Harris College of Nursing, ask me a series of questions regarding my perceptions of the roles and responsibilities of a professional nurse, and to independently assess the nursing care plans that I have written. I understand that the purpose of this study is to provide information about the perceptions and implementation of nursing roles by graduates from associate degree and baccalaureate programs. I understand also that the interviews will be privately conducted, taped for the convenience of data collection, and will last approximately one hour. I further understand that as a participant in this study there are no foreseeable risks.

I understand my responses will be kept confidential and every precaution will be taken to safeguard my anonymity as well as the anonymity of the patients served by my care plans.

I understand I will not be compensated for my participation, but that I may contact Ms. Glidewell by calling _____ if I have any questions before or after the interview.

I also understand that my participation is voluntary, that I may withdraw at any time, and that I may have access to the findings of the investigation upon request.

_____	_____
Date	Signature
_____	_____
Date	Debra Glidewell, Investigator
_____	_____
Date	Nancy C. Sayner, R.N., D.N.Sc.
	Supervising Professor
	Texas Christian University
	Harris College of Nursing

SAMPLE RESEARCH ABSTRACT (SHORT FORM)

PATERNAL EXPERIENCE DURING HOSPITALIZATION OF HIGH-RISK NEONATES

Supervising Professor: Patricia Newcomb
Dr. Nancy Sayner   Nursing Student

Sophisticated biomedical technology has made it possible to save the lives of ever smaller and sicker newborn infants. As a result intensive care nurseries are expanding their facilities at a rapid rate, and the number of families affected by the dramatic treatment of high-risk newborns grows daily. The experience of entrusting one's newborn child to the intensive care milieu of the hospital is unique and stressful. The purpose of this study is to explore the impact of this unique experience on fathers.

The study was composed of a series of twelve nonstructured interviews with fathers of hospitalized newborns. Continuous comparative analysis was the method used to extract dominant themes and processes from the data. Issues that appeared significant included the often-described period of shock and disorganization after the birth, infant comparisons, and efforts to "normalize" babies initially perceived as abnormal, paternal perception of role and responsibility, blaming, feeling of being cheated, and the importance of the hospital-family-kin-friend support system.

SAMPLE RESEARCH
ABSTRACT (LONG FORM)

THE PATIENTS' PASSAGE OF DECISION IN STROKE PREVENTION ABSTRACT

The purpose of this study was to gain a greater comprehension of the decision-making process as perceived and experienced by patients undergoing a selected surgical procedure for the prevention of stroke. Stroke is the third leading cause of death and disability in the United States. The major disease entity responsible for this statistic is cerebrovascular occlusive disease, which accounts for 80 percent of the 450,000 new strokes that occur each year. One surgical procedure presently being used for the prevention of progressive neurological deterioration and stroke associated with cerebrovascular occlusive disease is microvascular neurosurgical bypass. Patients found to be clinically qualified to undergo this intracranial bypass procedure are subsequently confronted with the decision to have surgery or not to have surgery. Basic to this decision is the component of prevention and the role of the patient in decisions that affect his or her health care.

The methodology used for this study was a field research method with interviewing being the primary research tool. Analysis of data was accomplished through the constant comparative method in conjunction with the generation of grounded theory advanced by Glaser and Strauss.

A sample of convenience consisting of fifteen adult patients was obtained. This sample represented 12 percent of the total patients who had bypass procedures performed by the neurosurgeon during the study. To gain a variance in perspective of the patients' decision-making a sample of convenience numbering seven family members or significant others was additionally secured.

Findings indicate that the patients' process of decision cannot be studied as a separate entity but only in the context of the decision. The decision process was found to comprise a series of interrelated and progressive phases based upon specific components that influence the decision. The goal to which the process of decision is directed is "quality of life." The phases of the decision process identified were: threat, trust, holding, contemplation, and compliance. The basis from which the process of decision evolves are four major influential components of decision: brain symptomatology, timetable, physician dyad, and family or significant other. As a result of the similarity discovered among the phases of the decision process and the major components influencing the decision, a conceptual model, "the patients' passage of decision in stroke prevention," was developed. This model provides a means of viewing decision making from the patients' perspective and offers the health professional a framework for developing individualized health care plans for patients confronted with the decision to undergo bypass surgery for the prevention of stroke. The model, in addition, has potential value in its application to other forms of preventative surgery. Although information consistent with the requirements of informed consent could be identified by the patient respondents of this research, it was not found to be among the major influential components of their decision.

LIST OF SELECTED SOURCES OF FUNDING

Annual Register of Grant Support
Marquis Professional Publications
200 East Ohio Street
Chicago, Illinois 60611

Directory of Research Grants
William K. Wilson, ed.
The Oryx Press
2214 North Central at Encanto
Phoenix, Arizona 85004

Foundation Grants to Individuals
The Foundation Center
888 Seventh Avenue
New York, New York 10106

Directory of Foundation Aids to Women
Gail Ann Schlachter, ed.
ABC-CLIO, Inc.
Santa Barbara, California 93100

Sigma Theta Tau
1100 West Michigan
Indianapolis, Indiana 46223

Nursing Research Support Section
Nursing Research and Analysis Branch
Division of Nursing—Room 5C-09
5600 Fishers Lane
Rockville, Maryland 20857

American Nurses' Association
2420 Pershing Road
Kansas City, Missouri 64108

The Foundation Grants Index
The Foundation Center
888 Seventh Avenue
New York, New York 10106
Attention: Donna V. Dunlop

INDEX

INDEX